CHOLESTEROL
CONTROL
COOKERY

CHOLESTEROL CONTROL COOKERY

by Dorothy Tompkins Revell
Registered Dietitian,

R.D., ADA

BERKLEY BOOKS, NEW YORK

This Berkley book contains the complete
text of the original hardcover edition.
It has been completely reset in a typeface
designed for easy reading, and was printed
from new film.

CHOLESTEROL CONTROL COOKERY

A Berkley Book / published by arrangement with
Royal Publications, Inc.

PRINTING HISTORY
Royal Publications edition published 1961
Berkley edition / August 1973
Eleventh printing / July 1982

ISBN: 0-425-05947-2

A BERKLEY BOOK ® TM 757,375
Berkley Books are published by Berkley Publishing Corporation,
200 Madison Avenue, New York, New York 10016.
The name ''BERKLEY'' and the stylized ''B'' with design
are trademarks belonging to Berkley Publishing Corporation.
PRINTED IN THE UNITED STATES OF AMERICA

Contents

PREFACE   7

SUGGESTED DIETARY OUTLINE FOR FIVE TYPES OF HYPERLIPOPROTEINEMIA   14

FOODS USED FOR HIGH-POLYUNSATURATED FATTY ACID DIET FOR CHOLESTEROL LOWERING   17

CHOLESTEROL CONTENT OF FOODS   21

TRIGLYCERIDE DIET   51

RECIPES: 57
    APPETIZERS   57
    SOUPS   61
    BREADS   63
    SAUCES   69
    MEATS AND FISH AND POULTRY   74
    SALAD DRESSINGS   92
    SALADS   96
    CAKES   101
    FROSTINGS AND TOPPINGS   109
    DESSERTS   112
    VEGETABLES   124
    COOKIES   129
    SANDWICH FILLING SUGGESTIONS   136
    MISCELLANEOUS   137
    CHONO COOKERY   143
    CHOLESTEROL MEAL PLAN EXCHANGE LIST   151
    COMMON ARTIFICIAL SWEETENERS   155
    SUBSTITUTIONS   157

REFERENCES OF INTEREST (ABBREVIATED BIBLIOGRAPHY)   159

INDEX   161

Dedicated

to

Mary Margaret Harrington,

formerly

Head of the Dietetic Department,

Harper Hospital, Detroit, Michigan

Preface

Diet is not the whole answer to avoiding heart attacks but perhaps it can give us a postponement. Diet *is* one very important factor, and we know that the earlier you start on a proper diet the better. Perhaps by convincing parents that nutrition is relative to positive health, many of the health-related tragedies of old age can be prevented for the younger generation. But convincing people that the food they eat *can* make a difference in their health, their performance and in their general outlook on life is a problem. The ordinary citizen lacks any strong motive for adjusting his life to dietary change.

In 1961, The American Heart Association recommended that physicians prescribe a diet *moderate* in fat content with substitutions of poly-unsaturated fatty acids for individuals who were prone to coronary artery disease or who had had an arteriosclerotic heart attack or a stroke, for the purpose of preventing or reducing the possibility or recurrence of these diseases. In 1962, the American Medical Association also recommended modification of the *amount and type* of dietary fat for individuals with serum cholesterol over 280/100 ml. or triglycerides over 250/100 ml. and published plans for fat-controlled meals. Current recommendations, to seek control of factors enhancing risk for patients with established coronary disease, have been broadened to include coronary-prone individuals and family groups. *Diet Recommendations* include reduction of the intakes of saturated fat, dietary cholesterol, simple sugars and the increased proportions of poly-unsaturated essential fatty acids. The medical boards of Norway, Sweden and Finland made similar recommendations for their whole populations. The American Heart Association indicated that 3–4 tablespoons of oil be included in the meal plan for the 2,000 calorie diet. The oil should be high in linoleic acid and taken daily as in salad dressing or incorporated into the diet pattern as desired.

There is a group of high molecular weight alcohols or sterols with solubilities similar to those of fat and for this reason are classified with the fats or lipids. The sterols in nutrition can be from animal or plant life. The sterol of greatest significance in food is cholesterol. Plant sterols are so poorly absorbed by the intestinal tract that their ingestion does not add to the blood. Plant sterols in the diet, besides not being absorbed, have the capacity to inhibit or block the absorption of cholesterol and may be regarded as therapeutic substances for the treatment of hypercholesteremia. Sterol accumulations come from two sources—the diet and those produced by the liver and intestine. Cholesterol is apparently synthesized at a relatively constant rate in man, and synthesis is not greatly affected by dietary cholesterol. The most direct way to affect the input of cholesterol is to limit the consumption of food rich in cholesterol. The cholesterol consumed in the human diet is now known to have a great effect on serum cholesterol levels. Recommendations for the treatment of hypercholesteremia and atherosclerosis do include methods for the restriction of cholesterol-rich foods in the diet. (Connor, M.D., University Hospitals of Iowa, ADA Journal March 1968).

Diets are being ordered with reference to the hyperlipoproteinemia as type 1, 2, 3, 4, 5. Some refer to these as the Fredrickson grouping. Booklets for each type are available for patient use from the Heart Information, National Heart and Lung Institute, National Institute of Health, Bethesda, Maryland 20014. The lipid profile reading can be the key to the diet order. Diets may be ordered for lowering the cholesterol, the triglycerides, the phospholipids respectively or in combinations.

Guidelines are needed for the choice of fat-containing foods in constructing such diets for the reduction of blood lipids. The nutrient components should be ones most effective in this reduction on one hand, and yet palatable, practical and acceptable on the other hand, since it is of long-term nutritional benefit. Proper foods for fat-controlled diets need to be chosen with knowledge not only of the amount of fat they contain but also their fat composition which in turn affects the fat composition of the diet. Emphasis is placed on dietary fats as to quality and quantity, total calories and dietary cholesterol. An effective diet breaks down because of (1) improper selection of animal products, (2) poor choice of vegetable oils and margarines and (3) insufficient amount of proper vegetable oils and their products.

1. It is not enough to tell a patient to reduce the animal fat in the diet. Animal products, chocolate and coconut are high in saturated fat and low in poly-unsaturated fatty acids. The seafood and glandular organs are high in dietary cholesterol and low in fat. Most fish is high in poly-unsaturated fatty acids and is a good meat substitute. Poultry is also low in fat. In an effective diet, animal

products are selected for their low-fat content and include a choice of lean beef, veal, lamb and pork. Further reduction of the saturated fat in the diet is made by avoidance of cream, whole milk, ice cream, bacon, animal fat, poultry skin, chocolate, coconut, butter, ordinary margarines, the Cheddar-type cheeses as they are made from whole milk, the egg yolk and the non-dairy cream substitutes, which are made from coconut oil. Patients are instructed to trim off the fat of the meat before cooking and after cooking.

2. The diet may become less effective because of poor choice of vegetable oils and their products. In this diet the poly-unsaturated fat is increased. Palm oils, such as coconut oil and cocoa butter, are high in saturates and low in the poly-unsaturates. Oils from fruits, seeds and grain are high in poly-unsaturates and low in saturates. Effective diets for serum cholesterol reduction contain safflower or corn oil and cottonseed oil. The safflower oil is the one with the highest percentage of the poly-unsaturated essential fatty acid, linoleic. Cottonseed and soy oil are the cheapest and most plentiful. Unfortunately, soy oil must be hydrogenated, and this process reduces the amount of the poly-unsaturated fatty acids and may increase the saturated fatty acids, depending on the extent of hydrogenation. The prescribed amount of oil can be used in baking, cooking and salad dressing. The heating of unsaturated fatty acids, as is necessary for the preparation of many foods, markedly decreases their unsaturations and safflower oil shows the least effect from the heat. For this reason the margarines and salad dressing in the diet are important because they are not subjected to heat. Eating less than the prescribed amount of the oil-containing foods will affect the diet.

3. An inadequate vegetable oil intake is one of the main reasons for failure to obtain significant serum cholesterol reduction. The amount of oil or its equivalent in food products for an effective diet depends on the calorie requirement of the individual. Five English walnut halves or

1 tablespoon of sunflower seeds or one-third ounce of sunflower seeds could be substituted for 1 teaspoon of safflower oil.

The dietary cholesterol content of the diet runs about 150–250 mg. per day. This can be controlled by the limited inclusion or exclusion of those foods rich in dietary cholesterol—for instance, egg yolk; glandular or organ meats, such as liver, sweetbreads, brain, heart, etc.; and shellfish or seafoods such as shrimp, lobster, crab, oysters, clams, etc. Morrison states the role of exogenous cholesterol appears to be as important as excess dietary fat. The spread used in the diet, such as margarine, can be made from safflower oil or corn oil and is obtainable in stick form or in a tub container at grocery stores.

In recent years, the importance of diet in the control of serum triglyceride has been emphasized. According to MacDonald of Guy's Hospital, London, if the high level of glyceride in the fasting serum is to be avoided because of its association with coronary thrombosis, then the dietary carbohydrate in the form of sucrose may be important when taken with a saturated fat. Kaufman and associates show that substitution of glucose for starch produces a marked increase of serum triglycerides similar to that caused by feeding sucrose. In a paper from the Department of Internal Medicine, University of Iowa, one statement of the summary on dietary carbohydrates reads "serum triglycerides were very responsive to the source of carbohydrates, rising with sucrose and falling with starch." In the diet used for triglyceride lowering, most of the monsaccharides and most of the disaccharides are eliminated from the diet; and the total carbohydrate for the day is approximately 125 grams or less. The carbohydrate for the day will come from the allowance of breads, cereals, potatoes or such substitutes as rice, the fruit and the milk allowances as well as the vegetables. Reference to the carbohydrate value of these items is indicated in the exchange list of foods on pages 151–152.

This is not a difficult diet to follow. Even those who

must select their food from a menu can meet the situation just as the diabetic patient is instructed to do. The big problem is to get the patient to accept the adjustment which has been indicated and to give him thorough instruction. The individual must understand the essential requirements. A Chinese proverb states: it is easier to make steel than to change peoples' ideas. Eating habits are deep-rooted and resistant to change. The question to be asked today is not "how do you change food habits" but "how do food habits change?"

Dorothy Revell, R. D.

Suggested Dietary Outline for Five Types of Hyperlipoproteinemia

HYPERLIPO-PROTEINEMIA*	TYPE 1	TYPE 2	TYPE 3	TYPE 4	TYPE 5
Sensitive to carbohydrate:	no	no	yes	yes	yes
fat:	yes	yes	yes	no	yes
Diet Is:	low fat, omit all fat	low dietary cholesterol poly-unsaturated fat increase	low dietary cholesterol 20% protein of calories 40% fat of calories 40% carbohydrate of calories	control carbohydrate 40% of calories moderate restriction of cholesterol	restrict fat to 25-30% control carbohydrate 50% moderate restriction of cholesterol
Calories in diet:	no restriction	no restriction	reduce weight, very important, if necessary high protein 75-125 gm. a day or 20% of calories	reduce weight, very important, if necessary not limited but for weight	reduce weight if necessary high protein 90-145 gm. a day, 24% of calories
Protein in diet:	total not limited but limit amount of lean cooked meat to 5 oz. for day	no limit best to be about 20% of calories			

14

Fat in diet:	Restrict to 25-35 gm. a day, the kind of fat not important. May use MCT, a special fat on the physician's order. Limit egg yolk to 3 per week (1 equals 1 oz. of cooked meat).	20-30 gm. of fat; saturated fat restricted; poly-unsaturated fat increased 30-45% of calories	control to 40% of calories, poly-unsaturated fat is preferred	low fat for weight control, poly-unsaturated fat preferred	restrict to 30% of calories, poly-unsaturated fat preferred
Dietary cholesterol:	not restricted	100 mg. daily. No egg yolk or glandular meats or shellfish. May have 9 oz. of lean meat a day (beef, lamb, pork, ham 3 oz. 3 times a week)	100 to 200 mg. a day	moderate restriction 300-500 mg. a day. May have 1 egg per week and glandular meats and shellfish once in a while	moderate restriction 300-500 mg. a day
Carbohydrate in diet:	not restricted	not restricted, 40% calories	no sugar, control and restrict 135-285 gm. a day	no sugar, control and restrict 135-285 gm. per day	no sugar, control and restrict 180-370 gm. (50%) per day
Alcohol in diet:	none	under physician discretion	under physician discretion	under physician discretion	none
Cholesterol, plasma:	elevated	elevated	elevated	normal or elevated	elevated
Triglycerides:	grossly elevated	normal or modestly elevated	usually elevated	elevated	elevated to markedly

15

* Thomas P. Sharkey, M.D., "Heart and Vascular Disease," *Journal American Dietetic Association*, vol. 58, April 1972, pages 340-342.

Foods Used for High Poly-unsaturated Fatty Acid Diet for Cholesterol Lowering

CHOLESTEROL LOWERING DIET

DIET PRINCIPLES

1. Reduction of the saturated fat in the diet. These fats can be hidden as the fat in the milk and the fat in the egg yolk as well as the solid or visible fat of the meat, the butter, the lard, etc. Coconut oil is also a saturated fat.

2. Inclusion of the poly-unsaturated fats rich in the poly-unsaturated essential fatty acids especially linoleic acid. Safflower oil and walnuts are high in the linoleic content.

3. Restriction of the dietary cholesterol by exclusion or limitation of the cholesterol rich foods as egg yolk, shell-

fish or seafood, and the organ or glandular meats as liver, sweetbreads, etc.

This diet is used when the blood cholesterol is elevated and the triglyceride is in the normal range.

FOOD	INCLUDED	EXCLUDED
Soups	fat free broth, consomme, skim milk soups	creamed soups
Vegetables	all types	creamed vegetables
Fruits	all types	none
Milk	skim, non-fat skim milk solids, buttermilk made from skim milk, skim milk yoghurt	whole, 2%, condensed, evaporated, whole milk yoghurt
Cheese	uncreamed cottage cheese, cheese made from skim milk, Cheez-ola* (a processed cheese made with corn oil)	cream cheese, cheese spreads, Cheddar cheese, cheese made from whole milk
Cream	none Poly-Perx* (a cream substitute made with corn oil)	sweet and sour cream, cream substitutes made with coconut oil
Desserts	ices, sherbet, ice milk, fruit whips	ice cream, puddings made with egg yolk and whole milk
Cereals	all types	none
Breads	most types	those made with a lot of egg yolk
Crackers	most types	cheese crackers
Nuts	especially walnuts; pecans, almonds, pistachio; old-fashioned peanut butter in small amounts (this is un-hydrogenated)	peanuts, cashews, Brazil, Macadamia, Coconut, hydrogenated peanut butter
Fats	unsaturated oils as corn, cottonseed, safflower, sesame seed, soybean, sunflower seed, walnut (these are rich in the poly-unsaturated essential fatty acid, linoleic acid). This is especially true of the safflower seed and walnut oils. Mayonnaise** made with oil mentioned above and without	olive oil, butter, lard, ordinary margarines, hydrogenated shortenings, pure mayonnaise, creamy type salad dressings, sandwich spreads, chicken fat, coconut oil, cocoa butter, peanut oil

FOOD	INCLUDED	EXCLUDED
	egg yolk. Soft type margarines made from the above oils.	
Meat	*very lean meats*—trim off all visible fat before cooking and after cooking; veal, venison, chicken, turkey, rabbit, dried beef, pheasant, game hen; beef as lean ground, steak or roast; lamb, pork, ham, goose, duck, Canadian bacon (back bacon)	meat fat, chicken fat, strip bacon, salt pork, corned beef, luncheon meats, sausages, liver, sweetbreads, glandular meats, poultry skin
Fish	all types of fish, such as tuna, pike, salmon, halibut, etc.	seafoods or shellfish, such as shrimp, crab, clam, lobster, oysters, caviar
Eggs	white of the egg. May have the whole egg (which is high in the dietary cholesterol content) *if* permitted by your physician. Chono*—this is an egg substitute.	egg yolk
Miscellaneous	flour, cornstarch, rice, grits, dried beans and peas, spaghetti, macaroni, noodles made without egg yolk, pickels, relishes, marmalade, jelly, jam, honey preserves, syrup, molasses, sugar, cocoa, gelatin, jello, condiments, herbs, seasonings, Angel food cake, tea, coffee, Sanka, Postum, wine, beer, liquor, candy (not chocolate), sauces made with skim milk, oil, or special margarine.	prepared cake and cookie and pudding mixes, Tom and Jerry batter, eggnogs, milk shakes, sponge (yellow) cake, egg sauces, such as Hollandaise, cream sauces, chocolate, meat gravies, candy made with cream, butter, chocolate, commercially fried potato chips, doughnuts, etc.

* Cheez-ola is available from Fisher Cheese Company, Wapakoneta, Ohio. Poly-Perx is available from Mitchell Foods, Inc., Fredonia, New York. Chono is available from General Mills, Chemical, Inc., Minneapolis, Minnesota.

** The mayonnaise used in some of these recipes is made according to instructions on page 92.

SUGGESTED MEAL PATTERN

BREAKFAST

	EXAMPLE
fruit or juice	orange juice
cereal	cornflakes
sugar	sugar for cereal
milk	skim milk for cereal
toast	toast
margarine	Chiffon margarine
beverage	coffee

NOON

soup	vegetable beef broth
sandwich	turkey sandwich
vegetables	lettuce, sliced tomatoes
salad dressing	1 tablespoon of safflower oil plus vinegar and desired seasonings
beverage	skim milk

MAIN MEAL

meat, fish, or poultry	roast beef, lean
potato or substitute	baked potato
vegetables, cooked	carrots
vegetables, raw	tossed salad
salad dressing	1 tablespoon of safflower oil plus vinegar and desired seasonings
bread	1 small dinner roll
margarine	Chiffon for the roll and vegetable
dessert	fresh fruit
beverage	tea

Note: It is very important that the 2 tablespoons of safflower oil be taken daily. If it is not desired at noon, then use the entire amount at the evening meal as the salad dressing. Some patients even take the oil with fruit juice or in skim milk or as is because of a dislike for salad dressings.

Cholesterol Content of Foods[1]

[1] Consumer and Food Economics, Research Division, Agricultural Research Service, U.S. Department of Agriculture, Hyattsville, Maryland. April 4, 1972.

| FOOD AND DESCRIPTION | HOUSEHOLD MEASURE UNIT AND/OR WEIGHT | CHOLESTEROL IN | | | FAT IN FOOD AS DESCRIBED |
		HOUSE-HOLD MEASURE MG.	100-GM. EDIBLE PORTION MG.	EDIBLE PORTION OF 1 LB. AS DESCRIBED MG.	%
Beef					
composite of retail cuts					
total edible					
raw					
with bone (refuse: bone, 15%)			68	261	*
without bone			68	307	*
cooked, bone removed	piece, approx. 4⅛ in. long, 2¼ in. wide, ½ in. thick or patty, approx. 3-in. diam. ⅝ in. thick; wt., 3 oz. (85 gm.)	(80)†	(94)	(426)	*
lean, trimmed of separable fat					
raw		(77)	65	295	‡
cooked	piece or patty (see item above); wt., 3 oz. (85 gm.)		(91)	(413)	‡
separable fat, raw	3 oz. (85 gm.)		75	340	#

22

Beef and vegetable stew cooked (home recipe, with lean beef chuck)	1 c. (245 gm.)	63	26	116	4.3
canned	1 c. (245 gm.)	36	14	66	3.1
Beef, dried, chipped, creamed	1 c. (245 gm.)	65	27	121	10.3
Beef potpie home-prepared, baked	piece, ⅓ of 9-in. diam. pie (210 gm.)	44	21	95	14.5
commercial, frozen, unheated	pie (216 gm.)	38	18	80	9.9
Brains, raw			>2,000	>9,000	8.6
Bread pudding with raisins	1 c. (265 gm.)	170	64	291	6.1
Butter regular (4 sticks/lb.)	1 Tbsp. or ⅛ stick (14 gm.)	35	250	1,134	81.0
	½ c. or 1 stick (113 gm.)	282			
whipped (6 sticks or 2, 8-oz. containers/lb.)	1 Tbsp. or ⅛ stick (9 gm.)	22	250	1,134	81.0
	½ c. or 1 stick (76 gm.)	190			

* Fat content of total edible portion of meat will vary, depending on the retail cut; however, cholesterol value is applicable to the total edible portion from all retail cuts.

† Numbers in parentheses denote imputed values.

‡ Fat content of the separable lean will vary, depending on the retail cut; however, cholesterol value is applicable to the separable lean portion from all retail cuts.

Fat content of the separable fat will vary depending on the retail cut; however, cholesterol value is applicable to the separable fat from all retail cuts.

FOOD AND DESCRIPTION	HOUSEHOLD MEASURE UNIT AND/OR WEIGHT	CHOLESTEROL IN HOUSEHOLD MEASURE MG.	CHOLESTEROL IN 100-GM. EDIBLE PORTION MG.	CHOLESTEROL IN EDIBLE PORTION OF 1 LB. AS DESCRIBED MG.	FAT IN FOOD AS DESCRIBED %
Buttermilk, fluid, cultured, made from nonfat fluid milk	1 c. (245 gm.)	5	2	10	0.1
Cakes					
baked from home recipes					
chocolate (devil's food), 2-layer, with chocolate frosting	piece, $\frac{1}{16}$ of 9-in. diam. cake (75 gm.)	32	43	196	16.4
fruitcake, dark	slice, $\frac{1}{30}$ of 8-in. loaf (15 gm.)	7	45	206	15.3
sponge	piece, $\frac{1}{12}$ of 10-in. diam. cake (66 gm.)	162	246	1,114	5.7
yellow, 2-layer, with chocolate frosting	piece, $\frac{1}{16}$ of 9-in. diam. cake (75 gm.)	33	44	197	13.0
baked from mixes					
angel food, made with water and flavorings	piece, $\frac{1}{12}$ of 10-in. diam. cake (53 gm.)	0	0	0	0.2
chocolate (devil's food), 2-layer, made with eggs, water, chocolate frosting	piece, $\frac{1}{16}$ of 9-in. diam. cake (69 gm.)	33	48	219	12.3
	cupcake, small, 2½ in. diam. (36 gm.)	17			

gingerbread, made with water	piece, 1/9 of 8-in. square cake (63 gm.)	trace	1	4	6.8
white, 2-layer, made with egg whites, water, chocolate frosting	piece, 1/16 of 9-in. diam. cake (71 gm.)	1	2	9	10.7
yellow, 2-layer, made with eggs, water, chocolate frosting	piece, 1/16 of 9-in. diam. cake (75 gm.)	36	48	210	11.3
Caviar, sturgeon, granular	1 Tbsp. (16 gm.)	>48	>300	>1,300	15.0
Cheeses, natural and processed; cheese foods; cheese spreads					
natural cheeses					
blue	1 oz. (28 gm.)	(24)	(87)	(395)	28.9
	1 c. crumbled (not packed) (135 gm.)	(117)			
brick	1 oz. (28 gm.)	(25)	(90)	(407)	29.8
Camembert	1 oz. (28 gm.)	(26)	(92)	(415)	25.0
	triangular piece, approx. 2¼ x 2⅛ x 2⅛ in., 1⅛ in. high; net wt., 1⅓ oz. (38 gm.)	(35)			
Cheddar, mild or sharp	1 oz. (28 gm.)	28	99	448	32.8
	1 c. shredded (113 gm.)	112			
Colby	1 oz. (28 gm.)	(27)	(96)	(437)	32.0
cottage (large or small curd) creamed					
1% fat	1 c. packed (267 gm.)	23	9	39	1.0
4% fat	1 c. packed (245 gm.)	48	19	88	4.2

| | | CHOLESTEROL IN | | | |
FOOD AND DESCRIPTION	HOUSEHOLD MEASURE — UNIT AND/OR WEIGHT	HOUSE-HOLD MEASURE MG.	100-GM. EDIBLE PORTION MG.	EDIBLE PORTION OF 1 LB. AS DESCRIBED MG.	FAT IN FOOD AS DESCRIBED %
Cheeses, continued					
uncreamed	1 c. packed (200 gm.)	13	7	30	0.4
cream cheese	1 Tbsp. (14 gm.)	16	111	504	35.2
	package, approx. 2⅞ x 2 x ⅞ in.; net wt., 3 oz. (85 gm.)	94			
Edam	1 oz. (28 gm.)	(29)	(102)	(465)	28.0
Limburger	1 oz. (28 gm.)	(28)	(98)	(447)	26.9
Mozzarella,	1 oz. (28 gm.)	(27)	(97)	(440)	26.5
low moisture part-skim	1 oz. (28 gm.)	18	66	298	16.8
Muenster	1 oz. (28 gm.)	(25)	(91)	(412)	30.2
Neufchatel	package, approx. 2⅞ x 2 x ⅞ in.; net wt., 3 oz. (85 gm.)	(64)	(76)	(344)	24.0
Parmesan grated	1 oz. (28 gm.)	(27)	(95)	(432)	26.0
	1 c. not packed (100 gm.)	(113)	(113)	(511)	30.8
Provolone	1 oz. (28 gm.)	(28)	(101)	(456)	27.5

Food	Measure				
Ricotta					
part-skim	1 oz. (28 gm.)	(14)	(51)	(232)	13.1
Swiss	1 oz. (28 gm.)	(9)	(32)	(145)	8.2
	slice, rectangular, approx. 7½ to 7¾ x 4 x 1/16 in.; wt., 1¼ oz. (35 gm.)	35	100	453	27.3
pasteurized process cheese					
American	slice, approx. 3½ x 3⅜ x ⅛ in.; wt., 1 oz. (28 gm.)	(25)	(90)	(410)	30.0
Swiss	slice, approx. 3½ x 3⅜ x ⅛ in.; wt., 1 oz. (28 gm.)	(26)	(93)	(423)	25.5
pasteurized process cheese food,					
American	1 Tbsp. (14 gm.)	(10)			
	slice, approx. 3½ x 3⅜ x ⅛ in.; wt., 1 oz. (28 gm.)	(20)	(72)	(328)	24.0
pasteurized process cheese spread,					
American	1 Tbsp. (14 gm.)	(9)			
	slice, approx. 2¾ x 2¼ x ¼ in.; wt., 1 oz. (28 gm.)	(18)	(64)	(292)	21.4
	1 c. shredded (packed) (113 gm.)	(73)			
Cheese sauce	1 c. (250 gm.)	44	18	80	13.6
Cheese soufflé, from home recipe	portion, ¼ of 7-in. diam. soufflé (110 gm.)	184	167	757	17.1

| | | CHOLESTEROL IN | | | FAT IN |
FOOD AND DESCRIPTION	HOUSEHOLD MEASURE UNIT AND/OR WEIGHT	HOUSE-HOLD MEASURE MG.	100-GM. EDIBLE PORTION MG.	EDIBLE PORTION OF 1 LB. AS DESCRIBED MG.	FOOD AS DESCRIBED %
Cheese straws	10 pieces, each 5 in. long, ⅜ in. wide, ⅜ in. high (60 gm.)	19	32	143	29.9
Chicken, all classes					
whole					
raw					
flesh, skin, and giblets (refuse: bones, 30%)			98	310	—
flesh and skin only			81	368	=
cooked, flesh and skin only	flesh and skin from 3-lb., ready-to-cook chicken, raw (624 gm.)	542	87	394	
cut-up parts					
breast					
raw (refuse: bones, 21%)			67	239	—
cooked					

total edible	meat and skin from ½ breast (from 3-lb., ready-to-cook chicken, raw) (92 gm.)	74	80	365	=
meat only	meat from ½ breast (from 3-lb., ready-to-cook chicken, raw) (80 gm.)	63	79	358	=
drumstick					
raw (refuse: bones, 40%)			88	239	‖
cooked					
total edible	meat and skin from 1 drumstick (from 3-lb., ready-to-cook chicken, raw) (52 gm.)	47	91	412	=
meat only	meat from 1 drumstick (from 3-lb., ready-to-cook chicken, raw) (43 gm.)	39	91	413	=
Chicken fat, raw			65	295	78.8
Chicken à la king, cooked, from home recipe	1 c. (245 gm.)	185	76	343	14.0

¶ Fat content of the edible portion as described will vary depending on the class; however, cholesterol value is applicable to the edible portion for all classes.

‖ Fat content of the cooked portion as described will vary depending on the class and method of cooking; however, cholesterol value is applicable to the cooked portion for all classes.

FOOD AND DESCRIPTION	HOUSEHOLD MEASURE UNIT AND/OR WEIGHT	CHOLESTEROL IN			FAT IN FOOD AS DESCRIBED
		HOUSEHOLD MEASURE MG.	100-GM. EDIBLE PORTION MG.	EDIBLE PORTION OF 1 LB. AS DESCRIBED MG.	%
Chicken fricassee, cooked from home recipe	1 c. (240 gm.)	96	40	182	9.3
Chicken potpie home-prepared, baked	piece, ⅓ of 9-in. diam. pie (232 gm.)	71	31	139	13.5
commercial, frozen, unheated	pie (227 gm.)	29	13	58	11.5
Chicken and noodles, cooked, from home recipe	1 c. (240 gm.)	96	40	182	7.7
Chop suey, with meat cooked, from home recipe	1 c. (250 gm.)	64	26	117	6.8
canned	3 oz. (85 gm.)	10	12	55	3.2
Chow mein, chicken (without noodles) cooked, from home recipe	1 c. (250 gm.)	77	31	140	4.0
canned	1 c. (250 gm.)	7	3	13	0.1
Clams** raw in shell soft (refuse: shell and	1 doz. large clams;	72	50	79	0.7

liquid, 65%)	14.4 oz. yielding approx. 5 oz. raw meat (143 gm.)	194	50	39	0.2
hard or round (refuse: shell and liquid, 83%)	1 doz. chowder clams; 5 lb. ⅔ oz. yielding approx. 13.7 oz. raw meat (389 gm.)	114	50	227	1.6
meat only	1 c. (19 large soft clams or 7 round chowders) (227 gm.)	(50)	(63)	(286)	2.5
canned, drained solids	½ c. (80 gm.)	51	129	583	15.0
fritters**	1 fritter (2-in. diam., 1¾ in. thick (40 gm.)				
Cod					
raw					
whole (refuse: head, tail, fins, entrails, scales, bones, and skin, 69%)	piece, approx. 5½ in. long, 1½ in. wide, ½ in. thick (80 gm.)	(66)	50	70	0.1
fresh only			50	227	0.3
dried, salted			(82)	(374)	0.7

** Cholesterol accounts for about 40% of the total sterol content of clams.

FOOD AND DESCRIPTION	HOUSEHOLD MEASURE	CHOLESTEROL IN HOUSEHOLD MEASURE	CHOLESTEROL IN 100-GM. EDIBLE PORTION	CHOLESTEROL IN EDIBLE PORTION OF 1 LB. AS DESCRIBED	FAT IN FOOD AS DESCRIBED
	UNIT AND/OR WEIGHT	MG.	MG.	MG.	%
Cookies					
brownies with nuts, baked from home recipe	1 brownie, approx. 1¾ x 1¾ x ⅞ in. (44 gm.)	17	83	378	31.3
ladyfingers	4 ladyfingers, approx. 3¼ x 1⅜ x 1⅛ in. (44 gm.)	157	356	1,616	7.8
Corn pudding	1 c. (245 gm.)	102	42	190	4.7
Cornbread					
baked from home recipe, made with degermed cornmeal	piece, approx. 2½ x 2½ x 1⅝ in. (83 gm.)	58	70	319	6.0
baked from mix, made with egg and milk	muffin, approx. 2⅜-in. diam. (40 gm.)	28	69	313	8.4
	piece, approx. 2½ x 2½ x 1⅜ in. (55 gm.)	38			

Crab, all kinds					
steamed in shell (refuse: shell, 52%) meat only	1 c. (125 gm.)	125	100	218	0.9
		125	100	454	1.9
canned, meat only	1 c. packed (160 gm.)	(161)	(101)	(456)	2.5
Crab, deviled††	1 c. (240 gm.)	244	102	460	9.4
Crab imperial‡‡	1 c. (220 gm.)	308	140	635	7.6
Cream					
half and half (cream and milk)	1 Tbsp. (15 gm.)	6			
	1 c. (242 gm.)	105	43	197	11.7
light, coffee, or table	1 Tbsp. (15 gm.)	10			
	1 c. (240 gm.)	158	66	299	18.0
sour	1 Tbsp. (12 gm.)	8			
	1 c. (230 gm.)	152	66	299	18.0
whipped topping (pressurized)	1 c. (60 gm.)	51	85	386	23.3
heavy whipping (unwhipped)	1 Tbsp. (15 gm.)	20			
	1 c. approx. 2 c. whipped (238 gm.)	316	133	603	36.7
Cream puffs with custard filling	1 cream puff, approx. 3½ in. diam., 2 in. high (130 gm.)	188	144	654	13.9
Custard, baked	1 c. (265 gm.)	278	105	476	5.5
Eggs, chicken					
whole					
raw or cooked with nothing added (refuse: shell, 11%)	large egg (50 gm.)	252	504	2,034	10.2
frozen, commercial	1 c. (515 gm.)	515	515	2,336	11.5

†† Prepared with bread cubes, margarine, parsley, eggs, lemon juice, and catsup.
‡‡ Prepared with margarine, flour, milk, onion, green pepper, eggs, and lemon juice.

| | | CHOLESTEROL IN | | | |
| | HOUSEHOLD MEASURE | HOUSE-HOLD MEASURE | 100-GM. EDIBLE PORTION | EDIBLE PORTION OF 1 LB. AS DESCRIBED | FAT IN FOOD AS DESCRIBED |
FOOD AND DESCRIPTION	UNIT AND/OR WEIGHT	MG.	MG.	MG.	%
Eggs, chicken continued					
dried, commercial			1,900	8,618	41.2
scrambled or omelet with milk and fat	omelet, prepared using 1 large egg (64 gm.)	263	411	1,864	12.9
whites, fresh, frozen and dried		trace	0	0	trace
yolks					
raw or cooked with nothing added	yolk from large egg (17 gm.)	252	1,480	6,713	30.6
frozen, commercial##			1,270	5,761	26.9
dried, commercial##			2,630	11,930	56.6
Flounder					
raw					
whole (refuse: head, tail, fins, skin, entrails, and bones, 67%)			50	75	0.3
flesh only			50	227	0.8
Frog legs, raw (refuse: bones, 35%)			50	147	0.2
Gizzard					
chicken, all classes					
raw			145	658	2.7

cooked	yield from 1 lb. raw, approx. 12½ oz. (354 gm.)	(690)	(195)	(884)	3.3
turkey, all classes					
raw	yield from 1 lb. raw, approx. 12¾ oz. (361 gm.)	827	145	658	7.3
cooked			229	1,039	8.6
Haddock					
raw	whole (refuse: head, tail, fins, bones, skin, and entrails, 52%)		60	131	trace
flesh only			60	272	0.1
Halibut					
raw	whole (refuse: head, tail, fins, entrails, scales, bones, and skin, 41%)		50	134	0.7
flesh only			50	227	1.2
cooked, flesh only, broiled with vegetable shortening	fillet, approx. 6½ in. long, 2½ in. wide, ⅜ in. thick (125 gm.)	(75)	(60)	(272)	7.0
Heart					
beef					
raw	1 c. chopped or diced pieces (145 gm.)	(398)	150	680	3.6
cooked			(274)	(1,245)	5.7

Includes small proportion of white.

35

| | | CHOLESTEROL IN | | | |
FOOD AND DESCRIPTION	HOUSEHOLD MEASURE UNIT AND/OR WEIGHT	HOUSE-HOLD MEASURE MG.	100-GM. EDIBLE PORTION MG.	EDIBLE PORTION OF 1 LB. AS DESCRIBED MG.	FAT IN FOOD AS DESCRIBED %
Chicken, all classes					
raw			170	771	6.0
cooked	1 c. chopped or diced pieces (145 gm.)	(335)	(231)	(1,049)	7.2
Turkey, all classes					
raw			150	680	11.2
cooked	1 c. chopped or diced pieces (145 gm.)	345	238	1,080	13.2
Herring					
raw					
whole (refuse: head, tail, fins, entrails, skin, and bones, 49%)			85	197	5.8
flesh only			85	386	11.3
canned, plain, solids and liquid	can, size 300 x 407 (No. 300); net wt., 15 oz. (425 gm.)	(412)	(97)	(440)	13.6
Ice cream					
regular, approx. 10% fat	1 c. (133 gm.)	53	40	181	10.6
	½ gal. (1,064 gm.)	426			

rich, approx. 16% fat	1 c. (148 gm.)	85	57	260	16.1
frozen custard or French ice cream	½ gal. (1,188 gm.)	682			
	1 c. (133 gm.)	97	73	331	10.8
	½ gal. (1,064 gm.)	777			
Ice milk					
hardened	1 c. (131 gm.)	26	20	92	5.1
	½ gal. (1,048 gm.)	213			
soft-serve	1 c. (175 gm.)	36	20	92	5.1
Kidneys					
all kinds (beef, calf, hog, lamb)					
raw	1 c. sliced pieces approx. ½ in. thick (140 gm.)	(1,125)	375	1,701	¶¶
cooked			(804)	(3,545)	¶¶
Lamb					
composite of retail cuts					
total edible					
raw					
with bone (refuse: bone, 16%)	2 pieces, approx. 4⅛ in. long, 2¼ in. wide, ¼ in. thick; wt., 3 oz. (85 gm.)	(83)	71	270	*
without bone			71	322	**
cooked, bone removed			(98)	(444)	

¶¶ Will vary, depending on kind.

| FOOD AND DESCRIPTION | HOUSEHOLD MEASURE UNIT AND/OR WEIGHT | CHOLESTEROL IN | | | FAT IN FOOD AS DESCRIBED |
		HOUSE-HOLD MEASURE MG.	100-GM. EDIBLE PORTION MG.	EDIBLE PORTION OF 1 LB. AS DESCRIBED MG.	%
Lamb, continued					
lean, trimmed of separable fat					
raw					‡
cooked	2 pieces (see item above); wt, 3 oz. (85 gm.)	(85)	70 (100)	318 (454)	‡
separable fat, raw	1 c. (205 gm.)	195	75	340	#
Lard			95	431	100.0
Liver					
including beef, calf, hog, and lamb					
raw	slice, approx. 6½ in. long, 2⅜ in. wide, ⅜ in. thick; wt., 3 oz. (85 gm.)	(372)	300 (438)	1,361 (1,987)	¶¶
cooked					¶¶
chicken, all classes					
raw	liver, approx. 2 in. long, 2 in. wide, ⅝ in. thick (25 gm.)	(187)	555 (746)	2,517 (3,386)	3.7
cooked					4.4

Food	Measure				
turkey, all classes					
raw			435	1,973	4.0
cooked			599	2,717	4.8
Lobster, cooked, meat only	1 c. chopped (140 gm.)	839	85	386	1.5
	1 c. cut in ½-in. cubes (145 gm.)	123			
Lobster Newburg‖ ‖	1 c. (250 gm.)	456	182	828	10.6
Macaroni and cheese, baked, made from home recipe	1 c. (200 gm.)	42	21	95	11.1
Mackerel					
raw					
whole (refuse: head, tail, fins, bones, skin, and entrails, 46%)			95	233	6.6
flesh only			95	431	12.2
canned, solids and liquid	can, size 300 x 407 (No. 300); net wt, 15 oz. (425 gm.)	(399)	(94)	(426)	11.1
cooked, flesh only, broiled with vegetable shortening	fillet, approx. 8½ in. long, 2½ in. wide, ½ in. thick (105 gm.)	(106)	(101)	(459)	15.8
Margarine					
all vegetable fat	1 Tbsp. or ⅛ stick (14 gm.)	7	0	0	81.0
⅔ animal fat, ⅓ vegetable fat	½ c. or 1 stick (113 gm.)	56	50	227	81.0

‖ ‖ Prepared with butter, egg yolks, sherry, and cream.

| FOOD AND DESCRIPTION | HOUSEHOLD MEASURE UNIT AND/OR WEIGHT | CHOLESTEROL IN | | | FAT IN FOOD AS DESCRIBED |
		HOUSE-HOLD MEASURE MG.	100-GM. EDIBLE PORTION MG.	EDIBLE PORTION OF 1 LB. AS DESCRIBED MG.	%
Milk					
fluid					
whole	1 c. (244 gm.)	34	14	64	3.5
low fat					
1% fat with 1 to 2% nonfat milk solids added	1 c. (246 gm.)	14	6	25	1.0
2% fat with 1 to 2% nonfat milk solids added	1 c. (246 gm.)	22	9	41	2.0
nonfat (skim)	1 c. (245 gm.)	5	2	10	0.1
canned, concentrated, undiluted					
evaporated, unsweetened	1 c. (252 gm.)	79	31	142	7.9
condensed, sweetened	1 c. (306 gm.)	105	34	156	8.7
dry					
whole, instant	1¾ c. (120 gm.)***	131	109	494	27.5
nonfat, instant	1⅓ c. low-density or ⅞ c. high-density (91 gm.)***	20	22	100	0.7
chocolate beverages					
commercial					
chocolate-flavored milk drink	1 c. (250 gm.)	20	8	36	2.3

40

with 2% added butterfat

chocolate-flavored milk homemade	1 c. (250 gm.)	32	13	59	3.4
hot chocolate	1 c. (250 gm.)	31	12	5€	5.0
hot cocoa	1 c. (250 gm.)	35	14	64	4.6
Muffins, plain, baked from home recipe	muffin, approx. 3-in. diam. (40 gm.)	21	53	24‡	10.1
Noodles whole egg dry form	package, net wt, 8 oz. (227 gm.)	213	94	426	4.6
cooked	1 c. (160 gm.)	50	31	141	1.5
chow mein, canned	1 c. (45 gm.)	5	12	54	23.5
Oysters††† raw in shell, Eastern, select (medium) size (refuse: shell and liquor, 90%)	12 oysters, about 4 lb.; yielding about 6⅔ oz. meat (180 gm.)	90	50	23	0.2
meat only, Eastern and Pacific	1 c., approx. 13–19 Eastern selects (medium); 19–31 Eastern standards (small); 4–6 Pacific medium; or 6–9 Pacific small (240 gm.)	120	50	227	2.0
canned, solids and liquid	3 oz. (85 gm.)	(38)	(45)	(203)	2.2

*** Amount needed for reconstitution to 1 qt.
††† Cholesterol accounts for about 40% of total sterol of oysters.

FOOD AND DESCRIPTION	HOUSEHOLD MEASURE UNIT AND/OR WEIGHT	CHOLESTEROL IN			FAT IN FOOD AS DESCRIBED
		HOUSE-HOLD MEASURE MG.	100-GM. EDIBLE PORTION MG.	EDIBLE PORTION OF 1 LB. AS DESCRIBED MG.	%
Oyster stew, home prepared†††					
1 part oysters to 2 parts milk by volume	1 c. (240 gm.)	63	26	120	6.4
1 part oysters to 3 parts milk by volume	1 c. (240 gm.)	57	24	108	5.3
Pancakes, baked from mix, made with egg and milk	cake, 6-in. diam., ½ in. thick (yield from approx. 7 Tbsp. batter) (73 gm.)	54	74	335	7.3
Pepper, sweet, stuffed with beef and crumbs	pepper, approx. 2¾ in. long, 2½-in. diam., with 1⅛ c. stuffing (185 gm.)	56	30	137	5.5
Pies, baked					
apple	sector, ⅛ of 9-in. diam. pie (114 gm.)	120	0	0	11.1
custard			105	476	11.1
lemon chiffon	sector, ⅛ of 9-in. diam. pie (81 gm.)	137	169	768	12.6

lemon meringue	sector, 1/8 of 9-in. diam. pie (105 gm.)	98	93	422	10.2
peach	sector, 1/8 of 9-in. diam. pie (114 gm.)	70	0	0	10.7
pumpkin			61	278	11.2
Popovers, baked from home recipe	1 popover, approx. 2 3/4-in. diam. at top (yield from 1/4 c. batter) (40 gm.)	59	147	665	9.2
Pork					
composite of lean retail cuts					
total edible					
raw					
with bone and skin (refuse: bone and skin, 18%)			62	232	*
without bone and skin					
cooked, bone removed	2 pieces, approx. 4 1/8 in. long, 2 1/4 in. wide, 1/4 in. thick; wt., 3 oz. (85 gm.)	(76)	62 (89)	283 (405)	**
lean, trimmed of separable fat					
raw	2 pieces (see item above); wt., 3 oz. (85 gm.)	(75)	60 (88)	272 (399)	‡
cooked					‡
separable fat, raw			70	318	#

43

| | CHOLESTEROL IN | | | |
FOOD AND DESCRIPTION	HOUSEHOLD MEASURE UNIT AND/OR WEIGHT	HOUSE-HOLD MEASURE MG.	100-GM. EDIBLE PORTION MG.	EDIBLE PORTION OF 1 LB. AS DESCRIBED MG.	FAT IN FOOD AS DESCRIBED %
Potatoes					
au gratin, made with milk and cheese	1 c. (245 gm.)	36	15	68	7.9
scalloped, made with milk	1 c. (245 gm.)	14	6	25	3.9
Potato salad from home recipe made with mayonnaise and hard-cooked eggs	1 c. (250 gm.)	162	65	293	9.2
Puddings, cooked					
chocolate, made from mix	1 c. (260 gm.)	30	12	53	3.0
vanilla (blanc mange) made from home recipe	1 c. (255 gm.)	35	14	63	3.9
Rabbit, domesticated, flesh only					
raw	1 c. chopped or diced (140 gm.)	(127)	65	295	8.0
cooked			(91)	(411)	10.1
Rice pudding with raisins	1 c. (265 gm.)	29	11	49	3.1
Roe, salmon, raw	1 oz. (28 gm.)	101	360	1,633	10.4
Salad dressings					
mayonnaise, commercial	1 Tbsp. (14 gm.)	10	70	318	79.9
	1 c. (220 gm.)	154			

salad dressing					
cooked, made from home recipe	1 Tbsp. (16 gm.)	12	74	337	9.9
	1 c. (255 gm.)	190			
mayonnaise-type, commercial	1 Tbsp. (15 gm.)	8	50	227	42.3
	1 c. (235 gm.)	118			
Salmon, sockeye or red					
raw					
steak (refuse: bone, 12%)			(35)	(141)	‡‡‡
flesh only	piece, approx. 6¾ in. long, 2½ in. wide, 1 in. thick (145 gm.)	(59)	(35)	(161)	†††
cooked, broiled with vegetable shortening, steak (refuse: bone, 12%)			(47)	(186)	6.5
canned, solids and liquid	can, size 301 x 411 (No. 1 tall); net wt., 16 oz. (454 gm.)	159	35	159	9.3
Sardines, canned in oil					
solids and liquid	can, size 405 x 301 x 014 (No. ¼ oil); net wt., 3¾ oz. (106 gm.)	(127)	(120)	(544)	24.4
drained solids	can (No. ¼ oil); drained wt., 3¼ oz. (92 gm.)	129	140	635	11.1
Sausage, frankfurter, all meat					
raw	1 frank, 8/lb. (56 gm.)	(34)	65	295	25.5
cooked			(62)	(279)	27.2

‡‡‡ No reliable data for fat content in sockeye (red) salmon.

		CHOLESTEROL IN			
		HOUSE-HOLD MEASURE	100-GM. EDIBLE PORTION	EDIBLE PORTION OF 1 LB. AS DESCRIBED	FAT IN FOOD AS DESCRIBED
FOOD AND DESCRIPTION	UNIT AND/OR WEIGHT	MG.	MG.	MG.	%
Scallops, muscle only¶¶¶					
raw			35	159	0.2
steamed	3 oz. (85 gm.)	(45)	(53)	(241)	1.4
Shrimp					
raw					
in shell (refuse: shell, 31%)			150	470	0.6
flesh only			150	680	0.8
canned, drained solids	1 c., approx. 22 large or 76 small (128 gm.)	192	150	680	1.1
Spaghetti with meat balls in tomato sauce					
cooked from home recipe	1 c. (248 gm.)	75	30	137	4.7
canned	1 c. (250 gm.)	39	9	41	4.1
Sweetbreads (thymus)					
raw			250	1,134	¶¶
cooked	3 oz. (85 gm.)	(396)	(466)	(2,114)	¶¶
Tapioca cream pudding	1 c. (165 gm.)	159	97	438	5.1
Tartar sauce, regular	1 Tbsp. (14 gm.)	7			
	1 c. (230 gm.)	118	51	233	57.8

Food	Measure				
Trout, raw, flesh only			55	249	11.4
Tuna, canned in oil, solids and liquid	can, size 307 x 113 (No. ½); chunk style; net wt., 6½ oz. (184 grm.)	(100)	(55)	(248)	20.5
drained solids	can (No. ½); chunk style; drained wt., 5½ oz. (157 grm.)	102	65	295	8.2
canned in water, solids and liquid	can, size 307 x 113 (No. ½); chunk style; net wt., 6½ oz. (184 grm.)	(116)	(63)	(287)	0.8
Turkey, all classes whole raw flesh, skin, and giblets (refuse: bone, 27%)			82	272	¶
flesh and skin only			74	336	¶
cooked flesh, skin, and giblets	flesh, skin and giblets from 13½-lb, ready-to-cook turkey, raw (3,680 grm.)	3,864	105	476	¶

¶¶¶ Cholesterol accounts for about 30% of total sterol of scallops.

FOOD AND DESCRIPTION	HOUSEHOLD MEASURE UNIT AND/OR WEIGHT	CHOLESTEROL IN			FAT IN FOOD AS DESCRIBED
		HOUSE-HOLD MEASURE MG.	100-GM. EDIBLE PORTION MG.	EDIBLE PORTION OF 1 LB. AS DESCRIBED MG.	%
Turkey, continued flesh and skin only	flesh and skin from 13½-lb., ready-to-cook turkey, raw (3,530 gm.)	3,283	93	422	=
light meat without skin					
raw	2 pieces, approx. 4 in. long, 2 in. wide, ¼ in. thick; wt., 3 oz. (85 gm.)	65	60	272	1.2
cooked			77	349	3.9
dark meat without skin					
raw	4 pieces, approx. 2½ in. long, 1⅝ in. wide, ¼ in. thick; wt., 3 oz. (85 gm.)	86	75	340	4.3
cooked			101	458	8.3
skin					
raw			110	499	42.0
cooked			127	576	39.2

Turkey potpie					
home prepared, baked	piece, ⅓ of 9-in. diam. pie (232 gm.)	71	31	139	13.5
commercial, frozen, unheated	pie; net wt., 8 oz. (227 gm.)	20	9	40	10.4
Veal					
composite of retail cuts					
total edible					
raw					
with bone (refuse: bone, 21%)			71	254	*
without bone	piece, approx. 2½ in. long, 2½ in. wide; ¾ in. thick; wt., 3 oz. (85 gm.)	(86)	71	322	**
cooked, bone removed			(101)	(457)	
lean, trimmed of separable fat					
raw	piece (see item above); wt., 3 oz. (85 gm.)	(84)	70	318	‡
cooked			(99)	(451)	‡
separable fat, raw			75	340	#
Waffles, baked from mix, made with egg and milk	1 waffle, 9 x 9 x ⅝ in. (yield from approx. 1⅛ c. batter) (200 gm.)	119	60	271	10.6
Welsh rarebit	1 c. (232 gm.)	71	31	139	13.6

FOOD AND DESCRIPTION	HOUSEHOLD MEASURE UNIT AND/OR WEIGHT	CHOLESTEROL IN				FAT IN FOOD AS DESCRIBED
		HOUSE-HOLD MEASURE MG.	100-GM. EDIBLE PORTION MG.	EDIBLE PORTION OF 1 LB. AS DESCRIBED MG.		%
White sauce						
thin	1 c. (250 gm.)	36	14	64		8.7
medium	1 c. (250 gm.)	33	13	59		12.5
thick	1 c. (250 gm.)	30	12	55		15.6
Yoghurt, made from fluid and dry nonfat milk						
plain or vanilla	carton; net wt., 8 oz. (227 gm.)	17	8	35		1.5
fruit-flavored (all kinds)	carton; net wt., 8 oz. (227 gm.)	15	7	30		1.2

50

Triglyceride Diet

TRIGLYCERIDE LOWERING

Some authorities distinguish two types of primary hypertriglyceridemia.[1]

1. One is due to the dietary fat, "fat-induced." The saturated fats of the diet cause a more prolonged rise in the triglyceride levels than do the unsaturated fats.
2. Another type results from endogenous fat synthesized from the dietary carbohydrate "carbohydrate-induced."

Monosaccharides and disaccharides are forms of carbohydrate and appear to raise the serum triglyceride to a greater degree than the carbohydrate "starch."

Monosaccharides are: glucose—fruits, sweet corn, corn syrup, honey; fructose—honey, fruits; and galactose—milk and milk products.

Disaccharides are: sucrose—molasses, cane and beet sugar, maple sugar, maple syrup; maltose—malt sugar,

[1] *Lipids in Nutrition*. Anderson Laboratories. Columbus, Ohio. 1962.

dextrin, malt products as beer; and lactose—milk and milk products.

The diet is generally used when the triglycerides of the blood are elevated and the serum cholesterol is in the desired range; however, it can also be used if the serum cholesterol level is elevated. The dietary recommendations include respect as to the quality and quantity of fat in the diet, along with the elimination of concentrated sweets and sugar and the restriction of the total carbohydrate content of the diet to approximately 135–370 gm. for the day.

TRIGLYCERIDE LOWERING DIET

This diet is to be used when the triglycerides of the blood are elevated and the cholesterol is in the desired range. The dietary recommendations include the elimination of concentrated sweets and sugar and the restriction of the total carbohydrate of the diet to approximately 135 gm daily.

The Carbohydrate allowed for the day may be selected from the following foods:

BREAD AND CEREALS
(YIELD 15 GM. CARBOHYDRATE IN
THE AMOUNT INDICATED)

1 slice of bread or 1 muffin or one small dinner roll or 1 biscuit
1 very small potato or ½ cup potato
½ cup of cooked rice, noodles, macaroni, spaghetti, lima beans
¼ cup of baked beans
¼ cup sweet potatoes
⅜ cup parsnips
½ cup cooked cereal as oatmeal or cream of wheat, etc.
¾ cup dry cereal as puffed rice or cornflakes, etc.
¼ cup grapenuts
2 graham crackers
3 soda crackers
5 saltine crackers
20 oyster crackers

FRUITS AND JUICES
(FRESH, DRIED, PACKED WITHOUT SUGAR; YIELD 10 GM. OF CARBOHYDRATE)

apple, 1 small
apple juice, ⅛ cup
applesauce ½ cup
apricots, fresh, 2 medium
apricots, dried, 4 halves
banana, ½ small
blueberries, ⅜ cup
berries, 1 cup
cantaloupe, ¼ of 6" diam.
cherries, 10 large or 15 small
dates, 2
figs, fresh, 2 large
figs, dried, 1 small
fruit cocktail, ½ cup
grapefruit, ½ small
grapefruit juice, ½ cup
grapes, 12

grape juice, ¼ cup
honeydew melon, ⅛ of 7" diam.
orange, 1 small
orange juice, ½ cup
papaya, ⅓ medium
peach, 1 medium
pear, 1 small
pineapple ring, 2 rings
pineapple juice, ⅓ cup
pineapple, crushed, ½ cup
plums or prunes, 2
prune juice, ¼ cup
raisins, 2 tablespoons
tangerine, 1 large
watermelon, 1 cup or 1½" thick
  of quarter slice

VEGETABLES (B)
(YIELD 7 GM. CARBOHYDRATE IN THE AMOUNT INDICATED: ½ CUP)

peas, beets, carrots, onions, pumpkin, turnips, rutabagas, winter squash

VEGETABLES (A)
(THESE MAY BE USED FREELY IN ANY AMOUNTS)

asparagus
broccoli
Brussels sprouts
cabbage
cauliflower
celery
chicory

cucumbers
eggplant
escarole
lettuce
mushrooms
okra

peppers
radishes
sauerkraut
string beans
summer squash
tomatoes & juice

watercress
bean sprouts
greens: kale, beet
spinach, collard
mustard, turnip
dandelion, chard

MILK
(YIELD 12 GM. CARBOHYDRATE IN THE AMOUNT INDICATED: 1 CUP = 8 OZ.

skim or buttermilk)

BEER
(12 OZ. YIELDS 16 GM. OF CARBOHYDRATE)

FOOD	INCLUDED	EXCLUDED
Soups	fat free broth and skim milk soups	creamed soups
Vegetables	all types—note carbohydrate allowance	creamed unless from milk allowance
Fruits	fresh, dried, frozen or canned without sugar—note carbohydrate allowance	sugar sweetened, fruit whips
Milk	skim, non-fat skim milk solids, buttermilk made from skim milk, skim milk yoghurt—note carbohydrate allowance	whole, 2%, condensed, evaporated, whole milk yoghurt
Cheese	creamed cottage cheese, cheese made from skim milk, Cheez-ola	cream cheese, cheese spreads, Cheddar cheese, cheese made from whole milk, cheese foods
Cream	none	all types and cream substitutes as these may contain sugar
Desserts	suggest the use of the fruit	ice cream, ice milk, fruit ices, sherbet
Cereals	most types—note carbohydrate allowance	sugar coated cereals
Breads	most types—note carbohydrate allowance	those made with a lot of egg yolk, frosted breads, sweet rolls
Crackers	most types—note carbohydrate allowance	cheese crackers
Nuts	especially walnuts; pecans, almonds, pistachio, old-fashioned peanut butter (unhydrogenated).	peanuts, cashews, Brazil, Macadamia, coconut, hydrogenated peanut butter
Fats	unsaturated oils, such as corn, cottonseed, safflower, sesame seed, soybean, sunflower seed, walnut (these are rich in the poly-unsaturated essential fatty acid, linoleic acid). This is especially true of the safflower seed and walnut oils. Mayonnaise* made with oil mentioned above and without egg yolk. Soft type margarine made from the above type of oils.	olive oil, butter, lard, ordinary margarines, hydrogenated shortenings, pure mayonnaise, creamy type salad dressing, sandwich spreads, chicken fat, coconut oil and cocoa butter, peanut oil

FOOD	INCLUDED	EXCLUDED
Meat	very lean meats, trim off the visible fat before cooking and after cooking; veal, venison, chicken, turkey, rabbit, dried beef, pheasant, game hen; beef as lean ground, steak, roast; lamb, pork, ham, goose, duck, Canadian bacon (back bacon)	meat fat, chicken fat, strip bacon, salt pork, corned beef, luncheon meats, sausages, liver, sweetbreads, glandular meats, poultry skin, breaded meats, fish or poultry
Fish	all types of fish, such as tuna, pike, salmon, halibut, sardines, etc.	seafoods and shellfish, such as shrimp, crab, clam, lobster, oysters, caviar, bread shellfish as French Fried shrimp, etc.
Eggs	white of the egg. May have the whole egg (which is high in the dietary cholesterol content) *if* permitted by your physician.	egg yolk
Miscellaneous	flour, cornstarch, sour pickles, condiments, relishes, gelatin, cocoa, seasonings, herbs, tea, coffee, Sanka, Postum, wine, beer, liquor in small amount if allowed by your physician; Dzerta gelatin, vinegar, lemon juice, catsup, mustard, cranberries; artificial sweeteners, such as Adolph's, Sweet Ten, Sweet-A, Sucaryl; may have olives.	prepared cake and cookie and pudding mixes, jam, jelly, honey, marmalade, preserves, syrup, molasses, Tom and Jerry batter, eggnogs, sponge cake (yellow), egg sauces as Hollandaise, cream sauces, alcoholic cocktails or drinks with sugar; pastries, cakes, cookies, chocolate, candy, sweet pickles, sugar sweetened beverages. *Sugar In Any Form.*
Potato or Substitute	white, yam, rice, noodles, etc.—note under the carbohydrate allowance	creamed or any milk added to the serving unless from the milk allowance

* The mayonnaise used in some of these recipes is listed on page 92.

SUGGESTED MEAL PATTERN

BREAKFAST	EXAMPLE	CARBO-HYDRATE GM.
fruit	½ cup of orange juice	10
meat	Canadian bacon	
toast	2 slices of toast	30
fat	margarine	
beverage	tea or coffee or Sanka	

NOON

soup	vegetable beef	
crackers	5 saltine crackers	15
meat, cheese, poultry	for a sandwich	
bread or bun	2 slices bread or 1 hamburger bun	30
fat	margarine	
vegetables (A)	lettuce, sliced tomatoes	
salad dressing	oil/vinegar salad dressing	
milk	1 cup	12

MAIN MEAL

meat, fish, poultry	roast beef	
potato	1 medium potato	30
vegetable (B)	½ cup cooked carrots	7
vegetable (A)	tossed salad	
salad dressing	oil/vinegar salad dressing	
fruit	½ serving = ½ pear	5
fat	margarine for vegetables	
beverage	tea or coffee or Sanka	

134 gm.

Recipes

APPETIZERS

MEAT SPREAD

1½ cup ground cooked
    liver

2 tablespoons lemon
    juice

1 teaspoon sage

2 tablespoons grated
    onion

2 teaspoons Worcester-
    shire Sauce

1 teaspoon unsaturated oil
    salt to taste

Mix the above ingredients well and serve with crackers.

TUNA CANAPÉS

1 tablespoon unsaturated
  oil
2 tablespoons grated onion
2 tablespoons mayonnaise*

1 teaspoon lemon juice
½ teaspoon dry mustard
  dash of garlic salt
1 teaspoon Worcester-
  shire Sauce
1 small can tuna fish

Rinse the tuna of the canned oil. Mix or grind all of the ingredients. Mold into shape desired and garnish with sliced stuffed olives and serve with thinly sliced rye bread. You may use the Waring Blender or a food grinder.

* See recipe under Salad Dressing.

SPICED PICKLED SHRIMP

Boil for 2 minutes 2 quarts of water, ½ cup chopped celery leaves, juice and rind of 1 lemon and 2 tablespoons pickling spices. Add 1 pound raw cleaned shrimp; bring to a boil and boil for 12 minutes. Drain immediately. Cool.

In a container put a layer of shrimp, then a layer of sliced onion (small green ones, if possible). Pour over this the following sauce:

1½ cups unsaturated oil
 ¾ cup vinegar
 ¼ teaspoon Tabasco
   Sauce
 2 tablespoons of capers
   and juice

1 teaspoon salt
1 teaspoon of Worcester-
  shire Sauce

This may be stored in the refrigerator for a week.

CRAB DIP

Make a sauce of 1 tablespoon of flour, 1 tablespoon un-saturated oil and 1 can tomato soup. When cool, add 1 tablespoon onion juice, ⅛ teaspoon of Tabasco Sauce and 1 can of rinsed and flaked crabmeat.

STUFFED EGG WHITES

Stuff the whites of boiled eggs with dry small curd cottage cheese mixed with mayonnaise and finely chopped walnuts.

BAC*OS COTTAGE CHEESE DIET DIP

⅓ cup skim milk
1 teaspoon lemon juice or vinegar
1 cup dry cottage cheese (large curd)

¼ cup safflower oil
½ teaspoon garlic salt, if desired
⅓ cup Bac*Os

Place milk, lemon juice, cottage cheese, oil and garlic salt in blender; blend 15 seconds. Scrape sides with rubber spatula. Blend about 1 minute longer or until smooth. Cover and refrigerate 3 to 4 hours. Just before serving, stir in Bac*Os.

BLENDER CHEESE DIP

1 cup uncreamed cottage cheese
¼ cup skim milk

2 tablespoons lemon juice
salt and pepper to taste

Combine ingredients in blender and blend until smooth. 1½ cup yield.

May add any desired seasonings or herbs.
May use as a "dip" with crackers, etc.
May use as a replacement for sour cream.
May use as a topping for vegetables, potatoes, etc.

GREEN ONION DIP

Blend 1 cup cottage cheese in blender with 2 tablespoons skim milk.

Variations: Add salt and pepper and chives to taste. Or add a commercial green onion dip mix to blended cottage cheese to taste. Delicious with vegetable frills.

CURRY DIP

1 cup cottage cheese blended in blender	2 teaspoons minced onion
2 teaspoons curry powder	½ teaspoon salt
½ teaspoon tabasco sauce	1 tablespoon lemon juice

Mix ingredients and serve. Yields 1 cup.

TUNA SPREAD

Mash one can of tuna fish thoroughly after the fish has been rinsed of the oil. Add ½ cup chopped olives, 1 teaspoonful of grated onion, ¼ teaspoon of lemon juice and enough mayonnaise* to moisten.

* Mayonnaise on page 92.

STUFFED CELERY STICKS

Stuff celery sticks with dry small curd cottage cheese blended with mayonnaise and grated onion. Sprinkle the tops with paprika. Finely chopped green or ripe olives may also be mixed with the cottage cheese.

COTTAGE CHEESE SPREAD

Add small amounts of skim milk to dry curd cottage cheese, using a food mixer or the Waring Blender, mix until well blended. Add salt and pepper or chives if desired. This spread can be used on sandwiches and crackers, also with fruit and tomato salads. The consistency will be as a thick spread.

SOUPS

CRAB SOUP

1 can tomato soup
1 can pea soup
½ cup sherry

1½ cups skim milk
1 can crab meat, flaked

Heat soups in a double boiler. Add the skim milk and crab meat and heat thoroughly. Add the sherry just before serving.

POTATO HAM CHOWDER

4 potatoes
2 tablespoons soft type margarine
¼ cup sliced green onions
½ cup chopped green pepper
2 cups water
1 teaspoon salt
⅛ teaspoon white pepper

¼ teaspoon paprika
3 tablespoons flour
2 cups skim milk
1 (12 oz.) can whole kernel corn
2 cups diced cooked ham trimmed of fat
chopped parsley

Peel and dice potatoes. In large saucepan melt margarine. Add onion and green pepper and cook until tender. Add potatoes, water and seasonings. Cover and simmer until potatoes are tender. Make a paste of flour and ⅓ cup water and add to the potato mixture. Add milk and cook until slightly thickened. Stir in undrained corn and diced ham. Heat through. Before serving, sprinkle with chopped parsley. Makes 6 servings.

FISH CHOWDER

3½ to 4 lbs. of haddock or cod, cut up
1 tablespoon soft margarine
1 medium onion, sliced
4 cups potatoes, diced
4 cups hot skim milk
1 tablespoon salt
⅛ teaspoon pepper

Place fish in saucepan and cover with 2 cups cold water. Cook until done. In a large pan melt the margarine, add the onions and cook slowly about 5 minutes. Pick fish from skin and bones. Add the fish stock and potatoes to the onions. Just enough water to cover the potatoes should be added. Boil until potatoes are nearly done, then add fish, hot milk, and seasonings. Simmer 10 minutes. Serve with crackers. Serves 8.

POTATO SOUP

2 cups skim milk
2 medium potatoes, cubed
¾ teaspoons of salt
dash of pepper
1 onion sliced & diced
1 stalk celery, diced
2 tablespoons unsaturated oil

hickory flavored suet

Add ingredients to skim milk. Cover and simmer for 20 minutes.

SPLIT PEA SOUP

2 cups of dried split peas
1½ quarts of water
1 onion, sliced and diced
4 branches celery, diced
½ teaspoon salt
⅛ teaspoon pepper
¾ teaspoon thyme
1 bay leaf

Soak peas overnight in 3 cups of water. Drain. Cook peas till tender in 1½ quarts of water to which has been added the celery, onion, salt, pepper, bay leaf and thyme.

Put soup through a sieve. Reheat and serve with crisp crackers.

CORN SOUP

1 can cream style corn put through sieve. Add the following:

1 teaspoon of grated onion
½ cup chopped celery
½ tablespoon of Worcestershire Sauce
1 pint of skim milk
1 tablespoon of flour
2 tablespoons of unsaturated oil

Blend the oil and flour, gradually add liquid and then the remaining ingredients. Heat thoroughly and serve.

VEGETABLE BOUILLON

4 cups tomatoes
1 stalk celery, chopped
2 carrots, chopped
2 sprigs parsley
¼ of a green pepper, chopped
1 bay leaf
2 teaspoons onion juice
salt and pepper to taste
1 wine glass sherry wine
2 cups water

Put tomatoes in a saucepan with the water, add all the vegetables and seasoning and let boil for 30 minutes. Strain. Add the sherry wine. Serve piping hot.

BREADS

BISCUITS I

2 cups flour (sifted)
3 teaspoons baking powder
1 teaspoon salt
4 tablespoons of unsaturated oil
⅔ cup of skim milk

Mix and sift dry ingredients together. Combine oil and milk. Pour all at once over the flour mixture. Mix with a fork and make into a soft dough. Knead lightly until smooth. Cut with small biscuit cutter and place on ungreased cooky sheet. Bake in hot oven 450 degrees for 12–15 minutes. 16 biscuits.

BISCUITS II

1¾ cups Gold Medal
    Flour
  3 teaspoons baking
    powder
  1 teaspoon salt

⅓ cup safflower oil
⅔ cup skim milk

Heat oven to 475 degrees. Mix dry ingredients in bowl. Pour oil and milk into measuring cup, but don't stir. Pour all at once into flour. Stir with fork until mixture cleans side of bowl and rounds up into ball. Smooth by kneading dough about 10 times without additional flour. With dough on waxed paper, press out ½ inch thick with hands or roll between sheets of waxed paper. Cut with unfloured biscuit cutter. Bake 10 to 12 minutes on ungreased baking sheet. Makes about 12 biscuits.

Drop Biscuits: Follow recipe above, except when mixture rounds into a ball, drop dough onto ungreased baking sheet.

Curry Biscuits: Add ¼ teaspoon curry powder to dry ingredients.

Chive Biscuits: Add ¼ cup chopped chives to dry ingredients.

Cornmeal Biscuits: Add ½ cup yellow cornmeal to the flour.

BUTTERMILK MUFFINS

2 cups flour
2 teaspoons baking
   powder
½ teaspoon salt
2 tablespoons sugar
2 egg whites, slightly
   beaten

1 cup buttermilk
½ teaspoon soda dissolved
   in 1 tablespoon water
2 tablespoons of unsatu-
   rated oil

Sift dry ingredients together. Add buttermilk, oil, slightly beaten egg whites and soda water. Mix lightly. Grease muffin tins. Bake 20 minutes at 400 degrees.

CARROT-ORANGE BREAD

1 cup sugar
1½ cups flour, sifted
1 teaspoon soda
½ teaspoon salt
1 teaspoon cinnamon
1 teaspoon baking
   powder

2 egg whites, slightly
   beaten
½ cup orange juice
4 tablespoons unsaturated
   oil
1 cup grated carrots
½ cup chopped nuts

Sift thoroughly dry ingredients, add nuts and carrots. To beaten egg whites add the oil and orange juice. Fold into the dry mixture. Pour into a wax-paper lined loaf pan. Bake 350 degrees about 50–60 minutes.

WHITE CORN BREAD

1¼ cups white corn meal
1¼ cups flour, sifted
4 teaspoons baking
   powder
1 teaspoon salt
¼ cup sugar

1⅓ cups skim milk
3 egg whites, slightly
   beaten
3 tablespoons unsatu-
   rated oil

Sift together the dry ingredients. Gradually add the milk. To beaten egg whites add the oil. Fold egg whites into the first mixture. Pour into a wax-paper lined loaf pan and bake 350 degrees for about 50 minutes or in a 9-inch square pan and bake 400 for 25–30 minutes.

SPICY TWISTS

1½ cups sifted flour
1 teaspoon dry mustard
½ teaspoon baking powder
½ teaspoon salt
    dash cayenne (optional)
5 tablespoons unsaturated oil
¼ teaspoon Tabasco Sauce
⅓ cup cold water
2 tablespoons flour
2 teaspoons paprika

Sift together 1½ cups flower, mustard, baking powder, salt, and cayenne. Add oil and Tabasco Sauce to water and sprinkle, one tablespoon at a time, over the ingredients, gently mixing and pressing with a fork until the dough just holds together. Combine 2 tablespoons flour and paprika. Sprinkle on a long sheet of waxed paper. Place dough atop the paper; roll in a 10 x 15 inch rectangle; turn to cover other side with paprika mixture. Cut in half lengthwise, then crosswise in ¾ inch strips. Twist each strip 2 or 3 times; place on ungreased baking sheet, pressing down ends of strips. Bake in 450 degree oven about 10 minutes, or till crisp and lightly brown. These are excellent with soup and salads. Makes about 3½ dozen.

OATMEAL BREAD

4 cups boiling water
2 cups rolled oats
2 tablespoons soft margarine or unsaturated oil
⅔ cup molasses
1 tablespoon salt
1 cake compressed yeast
½ cup lukewarm water
9 to 10 cups flour, sifted

Pour boiling water over rolled oats and margarine, cover and let stand one hour. Add molasses, salt and yeast cake (dissolved in lukewarm water). Add flour, gradually, beating it in with a knife. Let rise until double its bulk; cut down, shape into loaves and let rise again. Press into buttered bread tins; let rise again and bake 40–45 minutes in a moderate oven (350 degrees). Makes 4 loaves.

GRAHAM BREAD

1½ cups skim milk soured
   by the addition of
   1½ tablespoons of
   vinegar
2 tablespoons melted
   soft margarine
⅔ cup molasses and maple syrup (half of
   each or alone)

2 teaspoons baking soda
½ teaspoon salt
1⅓ cups graham flour
1⅓ cups flour, sifted
   raisins may be added

Mix in the order given. Bake in greased bread tins in a moderate oven (350 degrees) for 45–50 minutes.

PINEAPPLE BISCUITS

2 cups bread flour
2 teaspoons baking powder
1 teaspoon salt
2 tablespoons shortening

¾ cup skim milk
12 cubes of sugar
¼ cup pineapple juice

Mix and sift all dry ingredients except sugar. Blend in shortening with fork or fingers. Add milk gradually and mix with a table knife. Place on floured board and knead for one minute. Pat down and roll out lightly to ½ inch thickness. Cut out with biscuit cutter. Soak sugar cubes 30 seconds in pineapple juice. Make indentation in center of biscuit, place cube in it. A few drops of pineapple juice may also be placed in the indentation. Place on greased cookie sheet, bake 12 minutes at 450 degrees.

SWEET POTATO BISCUITS

¾ cup mashed sweet po-
    tatoes
4 tablespoons melted
    margarine

⅔ cup skim milk
1¼ cups flour
2 teaspoons baking
    powder

Add margarine to mashed sweet potatoes and then stir in milk. Sift dry ingredients together and then sift into sweet potato mixture. Roll it out ½ inch thick and cut with floured biscuit cutter. Place on greased sheet. Bake 450 degree oven for 15 minutes.

BREAKFAST PUFFS

⅓ cup safflower oil
½ cup sugar
1 egg white
1½ cups Gold Medal
    Flour
½ teaspoon soda
½ teaspoon cinnamon

½ teaspoon salt
¼ teaspoon nutmeg
½ cup buttermilk
1 egg white, beaten
3 tablespoons sugar

Heat oven to 350 degrees. Oil bottoms of muffin cups or use paper baking cups. Mix oil, ½ cup sugar and 1 egg white thoroughly. Stir together flour, soda, salt and nutmeg; stir into oil mixture alternately with buttermilk. Fill muffin cups ⅔ full. Bake 20–25 minutes. Remove muffins from cups; brush tops with beaten egg white. Mix 3 tablespoons sugar and the cinnamon; sprinkle ¼ teaspoon of mixture over each muffin. Serve immediately. Makes 12 puffs.

CINNAMON MUFFINS

2 cups sifted flour
3 teaspoons baking
  powder
2 tablespoons sugar
½ teaspoon salt

2 egg whites, slightly
  beaten
2 tablespoons unsaturated
  oil
1 cup skim milk

Mix and sift the dry ingredients. Add oil to milk and stir into the dry mixture. Fold in the egg whites. Drop into greased muffin pans or pour batter into an oiled cake pan 8 inches square. Sprinkle with ¼ cup sugar mixed with 1 teaspoon cinnamon. Bake at 425 degrees for about 20 minutes if muffin pans are used or at 375 degrees for about 30 minutes if cake pan is used.

SAUCES

BARBECUE SAUCE

1 large onion, chopped
1 green pepper, chopped
½ cup celery
3 tablespoons unsaturated
  oil
¾ cup water
3 tablespoons sugar

3 tablespoons vinegar
4 tablespoons lemon
  juice
1½ cups tomato catsup
1½ tablespoons Worces-
  tershire Sauce
1½ teaspoons dry mustard

Cook onion, pepper and celery slowly in the oil till tender. Add remaining ingredients and simmer 10 minutes.

LOW CALORIE LEMON SAUCE

2 tablespoons cornstarch
¼ teaspoon salt
1 cup hot water
½ teaspoon grated lemon
  peel

2 tablespoons lemon juice
non-caloric liquid sweet-
  ener equivalent to ¼
  cup sugar
1 drop yellow food color-
  ing

Stir cornstarch and salt together in small saucepan. Gradually stir in water. Cook, stirring constantly, until mixture thickens and boils. Boil and stir 1 minute. Remove from heat. Stir in remaining ingredients. Makes 1 cup.

BLUEBERRY SAUCE

1 lb. can water-packed blueberries or fresh blueberries	1 teaspoon lemon juice artificial sweetener to taste
2 teaspoons cornstarch	

Cook and stir blueberries and 2 teaspoons constarch until mixture thickens and bubbles. Add artificial sweetener and lemon juice. Makes 1 cup.

PORT SAUCE FOR MEAT

Reduce some port to half its amount. Add the same quantity of meat juice, a little lemon juice and shredded orange. Boil and thicken the sauce with cornstarch mixed with a little water. Reduce slightly. Then add raisins, blanched almonds, chopped red pepper (small amount), more shredded orange peel and more lemon juice according to desired taste.

BROWN GRAVY

Blend 4 tablespoons of unsaturated oil with 4 tablespoons of flour or 2 tablespoons of cornstarch. Add 2 cups of fat free broth.* Stir over direct heat until the gravy boils. Add ½ teaspoon of Kitchen Bouquet. Salt and pepper to taste.

* 2 bouillon cubes plus 2 cups of water may be used in place of the meat stock.

TARTAR SPREAD

¼ lb. unsaturated marga-
    rine spread
½ teaspoon lemon juice
1 teaspoon Worcester-
    shire Sauce
¼ teaspoon French
    mustard

1 tablespoon finely
    chopped parsley
dash of garlic powder
salt to taste

Cream the ingredients. Spread on rounds of dark bread and decorate with anchovy. Try a dab on broiled meat just before serving or on baked potato which has been slashed and pressed open.

WHITE SAUCE

2 tablespoons flour
¼ teaspoon salt
    dash pepper

1 tablespoon unsaturated
    oil
1 cup skim milk

Combine flour, salt, pepper. Add the oil to the milk. Slowly add liquid to the dry ingredients. Cook over a low heat until thickened. Stirring constantly. Makes about 1 cup of sauce.

BOURBON MARINADE FOR BEEF

¼ cup safflower oil
¼ cup bourbon
2 tablespoons soy sauce
1 teaspoon Worcestershire
    sauce

1 teaspoon garlic powder
freshly ground pepper

Place all ingredients in a blender and blend well. Pour over meat (rump or chuck roast) and leave at room temperature for two days. Turn meat and baste it several times each day. Broil meat over charcoal to desired doneness, basting with marinade during cooking.

CUSTARD SAUCE

1 envelope low calorie
  vanilla pudding
2½ cups skim milk

⅛ to ¼ teaspoon nutmeg,
  or 2 teaspoons rum
  extract

Place pudding mix in saucepan. Add ¼ cup milk. Stir until thoroughly blended. Add remaining milk and nutmeg. Cook and stir over medium heat until mixture comes to a boil. Chill. (Sauce thickens as it cools.) Before serving, stir or beat with rotary beater until creamy. Serve over canned fruits. Makes about 2½ cups.

SPAGHETTI SAUCE WITH MEAT

1 lb. lean ground beef
1 8 oz. can tomato sauce
1 lb. can tomatoes
2 tablespoons green pep-
  per
1 teaspoon mustard
  dash of oregano
¾ cup water

½ cup onion
¼ cup celery
salt and pepper to taste
1 tablespoon Worcester-
  shire Sauce
sugar substitute equal to
  1 teaspoon sugar, if
  desired

In a skillet break up ground hamburger, brown, and drain off excess fat. Add all other ingredients. Bring to a boil, reduce heat and simmer for 1 hour and 15 minutes. Serve over spaghetti.

SWEET-SOUR BAR-B-QUE SAUCE

½ cup soft type margarine
¼ teaspoon dry mustard
1 cup vinegar
1 onion, chopped
2 teaspoons Worcester-
  shire Sauce

1¼ cup chili sauce
2 teaspoons lemon juice
2 lemons sliced paper
  thin
½ teaspoon chili powder
1½ cups brown sugar

Combine and cook over low heat for 2 hours. Fine for beef, chicken or fish.

TERIYAKI SAUCE

For 2 lbs. of meat, chicken, pork, ribs, fish, etc. 2 tablespoons sugar, increase or decrease as desired. Combine 1 tablespoon grated fresh ginger root or powdered ginger, 1 clove garlic crushed with 1 cup soy sauce. Marinate meat in sauce one-half hour or brush sauce on meat before broiling or baking. Sauce will keep in the refrigerator.

MUSTARD MARINADE FOR BEEF

1 cup prepared mustard	2 tablespoons vinegar or
1¼ cup sherry	lemon juice
½ cup safflower oil	¼ cup catsup
2 teaspoons brown sugar	

Place all ingredients in blender and blend well. Pour over chuck roast and let stand at room temperature for two days. Turn meat and baste as needed to keep well coated. Broil meat to desired doneness. Onions may be sliced over meat and broiled with it.

FISH COCKTAIL SAUCE

½ cup tomato juice	½ teaspoon salt
1 teaspoon prepared horseradish	½ teaspoon finely chopped parsley
1 teaspoon lemon juice	any other seasoning desired
½ teaspoon Worcestershire Sauce	

Cook tomato juice down to half its volume. Mix additional ingredients with tomato juice. Serve with cooked fish.

BASIC CREAM SAUCE WITH
DRY SKIM MILK

2 tablespoons unsaturated
  oil
2 tablespoons flour
3 tablespoons dry skim
  milk

½ teaspoon salt
1 cup water or water in
  which vegetables were
  cooked

Mix flour, dry skim milk and salt. Add oil to the water
and blend this with the dry ingredients. Stir until well
mixed. Cook over low heat, stirring constantly until thick
and smooth. Yields about 1 cup.

MEATS AND FISH AND POULTRY

Note: When unsaturated oil is used to sauté meats, it
should *not* be allowed to reach the smoking point *nor* used
again.

BAKED SALMON

1 large can salmon
1 egg white, slightly
  beaten
4 soda crackers, crushed
⅓ cup skim milk

½ teaspoon salt
  pepper to taste
½ cup canned or fresh
  peas

Flake the salmon and add the remaining ingredients.
Mix and place in an oiled baking dish. Cover and bake at
325 degress for about 45 minutes. Serve with lemon slices.

OVEN-BAKED CHICKEN IN WINE

Cut chicken into serving pieces. After cleaning, place
the chicken in a baking pan and sprinkle with salt, pepper
and paprika. Add 6 teaspoons of white wine and 2 table-

spoons water. Cover. Bake at 325 degrees for 1 hour and 30 minutes. The cover may be removed the last 20 minutes to brown the chicken.

MEAT LOAF

2 lbs. lean ground beef
1 egg white, slightly
   beaten
2 teaspoons unsaturated
   oil
8 soda crackers, crushed
¼ cup catsup

¼ cup skim milk
¼ teaspoon oregano
¼ teaspoon poultry
   seasoning
1 teaspoon salt
¼ teaspoon pepper

Mix all the ingredients and place in baking pan. Diced onion and sliced tomato may be added to the loaf. Bake at 350 degrees for 1 hour. This is good as cold meat for slicing.

OVEN-BAKED SPANISH PORK CHOPS

Cut off all the fat from the pork chops. Place in shallow baking dish and cover with some of the sauce mixture. Turn frequently and add more liquid to keep covered.

Sauce:
4 tablespoons catsup
¼ cup vinegar
½ cup water

1 tablespoon Worcester-
   shire Sauce
¼ teaspoon mustard

Bake at 325 degrees for 1 hour and 30 minutes.

FISH FILLETS

I

Wash fish fillets and wipe with cloth. Chop celery, onion and parsley and brown in unsaturated oil till tender. Place these vegetables in a shallow baking dish. Put the fish fillets on top. Brush unsaturated oil over the fish and then sprinkle with salt, pepper, and paprika. Bake at 450 degrees for 30 minutes or until well browned. Serve with lemon slices.

II

Fish fillets are easily prepared by wrapping in aluminum foil. Wash fish, dry, place on sheet of foil. Sprinkle with salt, pepper, lemon juice and paprika. Fold edges of foil securely. Bake 450 degrees for about 25–30 minutes.

CRAB MEAT PANCAKES

1 small can crab meat, flaked and rinsed
1 raw carrot, shredded
½ cup celery, finely chopped
1 teaspoon grated onion
½ teaspoon salt
dash of pepper
2 egg whites, slightly beaten
3 tablespoons unsaturated oil

After flaking the crab meat, rinse under cold water and drain thoroughly. Heat 3 tablespoons of oil in a heavy frying pan. Mix the beaten egg whites with the remaining ingredients. Pour into the heated pan and cook over a low heat until pancake is well set. Cut into quarters and turn each quarter carefully. Serve at once. This is very good served with a tossed salad and a cup of tea for supper or company.

FISH AND NOODLES

1 can fish, flaked
2 cups cooked noodles
1 small onion, chopped
1 can tomatoes
salt and pepper
⅓ cup diced celery

Mix all ingredients and place in an oiled dish and bake at 350 degrees for 30 minutes.

VEAL OR CHICKEN À LA MARENGO

Cut chicken into desired serving pieces. Clean and wash.
Dry. Sprinkle with salt and pepper, dredge with flour and
sauté in unsaturated oil. Put in a stew pan, cover with
sauce and cook slowly until tender. Add ½ can mushrooms cut in pieces and cook 5 minutes. Arrange chicken
on serving dish and pour around the sauce; garnish with
parsley.

Sauce:

- 3 tablespoons unsaturated oil
- 1 tablespoon onion, chopped
- 1 carrot, chopped
- ½ cup diced celery
- ¼ cup flour
- 2 cups boiling water
- 1 teaspoon salt
- ½ cup stewed tomatoes
- dash of pepper

Sauté vegetables in oil. Add flour, salt and pepper and
cook until flour is brown. Add gradually the water and
tomato. Cook five minutes.

RED SNAPPER

- ¼ cup minced shallots or green onions
- 2 cups finely sliced onion (2 large)
- 1 can (1 lb., 12 oz.) tomatoes, coarsely chopped
- 1 lb. fresh okra, washed and sliced, or 2 packages (10 oz. each) frozen cut okra, thawed
- 6 fillets red snapper or striped bass (about 6 oz. each)
- salt and pepper
- Melted soft type margarine

Heat oven to 400 degrees. Grease a shallow baking pan just large enough to hold the fillets. Fold the fillets, if desired. Arrange shallots or green onions, onions, tomatoes and okra on bottom of pan. Sprinkle fillets with salt and pepper. Place fillets over vegetables. Brush with melted margarine. Bake 10 to 15 minutes or until fish flakes easily. Remove fillets with large slotted spatula. Keep warm. Transfer vegetables and juice to saucepan. Bring to a boil. Simmer 5 minutes. Correct seasoning to taste. Arrange vegetables in center of serving platter. Place fillets over vegetables. Pour remaining juice over fish. Makes 6 servings.

BRAISED FISH, PORTUGUESE

1 large onion, sliced
3 tablespoons safflower oil
½ teaspoon crumbled bay leaf
1 clove garlic, minced or mashed
1 large can (1 lb., 12 oz.) Italian-style, pear-shaped tomatoes
1 tablespoon chopped parsley

1 cup dry white wine (or ¼ cup lemon juice with ¾ cup water)
1 teaspoon salt
2 to 2½ pounds fish steaks or fillets (about ½ to ¾ inch thick)
chopped parsley for garnish
lemon wedges

In an 11 or 12 inch frying pan, sauté the onion in oil until soft. Add bay, garlic, tomatoes, parsley, wine, and salt. Simmer, uncovered, stirring occasionally and breaking up tomatoes, for about 15 minutes. Set in fish and simmer slowly, uncovered (spoon sauce over fish several times), until fish flakes when tested with a fork, about 12 to 15 minutes depending on fish used. Remove fish to a serving plate and keep warm. Boil sauce until reduced and thickened slightly; pour over fish. Sprinkle with parsley. Pass lemon wedges at the table. Makes about 6 servings.

BAKED FISH WITH PIQUANT SAUCE

2 to 3 lbs. thick (about 1 inch) fish steaks or fillets

1 teaspoon salt

2 tablespoons flour, approximately

2 medium sized onions, sliced

¼ cup safflower oil

⅓ cup white wine vinegar

3 cloves garlic, minced or mashed

1 teaspoon each oregano and prepared mustard

⅛ teaspoon powdered saffron (optional)

1 tablespoon each minced parsley and fresh coriander (or use 2 tablespoons parsley and ½ teaspoon ground coriander)

1 tablespoon lemon juice

About ¼ cup water or dry white wine

lemon wedges (optional)

Sprinkle fish with salt, then dust lightly all over with flour. Arrange fish in a shallow baking dish, about 8 x 12 inches. In a frying pan, sauté the onions in oil until limp, then distribute over fish. Combine wine vinegar, garlic, oregano, mustard, saffron (if used), parsley, coriander, and lemon juice; mix well and pour over fish. Pour water or wine around fish. Bake, uncovered, in a 350 degree oven until the fish flakes easily when tested with a fork, about 45 minutes. Add a little water if liquid cooks away. Serve with lemon if you wish. Makes about 6 servings.

CURRIED CHICKEN WITH PAPAYA

2½ lbs. chicken legs and thighs, approximately

3 tablespoons flour

1 teaspoon salt

⅛ teaspoon pepper

3 tablespoons safflower oil

1 large onion, chopped

1 tablespoon curry powder

1 cup chicken stock

2 tablespoons chopped candied ginger or ½ teaspoon ground ginger

1 papaya, peeled and cut lengthwise in thick slices

2 tablespoons lime juice

Wash the chicken and pat dry. Mix the flour, salt and pepper; dredge chicken in mixture to coat all over. Heat the oil in an 11 or 12 inch frying pan (one with a tight fitting lid) over medium high heat. Put in chicken pieces and shake any extra flour over top. Cook, turning until chicken is browned on all sides; remove from pan and set aside. Add onion to the pan and sauté until soft, about 4 minutes. Stir in curry powder and cook about 1 minute. Then stir in the chicken stock base and the ginger. Return chicken to pan, cover and simmer for 40 minutes or until meat loses any pinkness in the center of the thickest part. Garnish with papaya, then sprinkle lime juice over all. Makes about 4 servings.

BEEF STEW

1½ lbs. beef stew meat, cut in 1 inch cubes, trim off fat	⅓ cup dry red wine
	½ teaspoon anchovy paste
	1 clove garlic, minced
2 tablespoons safflower or corn oil	2 beef bouillon cubes
	1 small bay leaf
1 large apple, pared and shredded (1 cup)	⅛ teaspoon dried thyme, crushed
1 medium carrot, shredded (½ cup)	4 teaspoons cornstarch
	¼ cup cold water
½ onion, sliced	¼ teaspoon kitchen bouquet
½ cup water	

Brown meat in hot oil. Add apple, carrot, onion, the ½ cup water, the wine, anchovy paste, garlic, bouillon cubes, bay leaf and thyme. Cover and cook over low heat for 2 hours or till beef is tender. Remove bay leaf. Combine cornstarch and the ¼ cup cold water; add to beef mixture. Cook and stir till thickened. Stir in kitchen bouquet. Makes 4 servings.

INTERNATIONAL DATELINE CHICKEN

3 large chicken breasts cut in half
¼ cup soft type margarine
1 14 oz. can chicken broth
1 tablespoon minced onion
1 teaspoon salt
½ teaspoon curry powder
pepper to taste

1 11 oz. can mandarin oranges
2 tablespoons cornstarch
1 teaspoon lemon juice
1 cup thinly sliced green pepper
1 cup pitted dates cut in half

Wash chicken breasts, drain and pat dry. Melt margarine in skillet, cook chicken slowly in skillet to a golden brown. Combine broth, onion, salt, curry powder and pepper. Pour over chicken, cover and simmer for 45 minutes or until chicken is fork tender. Remove chicken to a warm platter and keep warm. Drain oranges, reserving syrup. Combine syrup, cornstarch, lemon juice and stir into brown pan juices. Cook, stirring constantly until thick and clear. Add green pepper and dates, simmer 3 to 4 minutes and add orange sections. Serve hot over chicken breasts. Serves 6.

CHICKEN JUBILEE

3 two lb. chickens, halved or split
paprika
1 teaspoon salt
6 tablespoons soft type margarine
1 tablespoon flour
1 teaspoon sugar
⅛ teaspoon ground allspice
⅛ teaspoon ground cinnamon

⅛ teaspoon mustard
2 cups canned pitted cherries water packed
1 cup crushed pineapple
1 chicken bouillon cube
2 tablespoons dark rum (or Chablis and more liquid)
¼ teaspoon red food color

Season chicken with paprika and salt. Sauté in margarine and brown. Blend flour, sugar, spices and add to chicken. Drain cherries and pour liquid over chicken. Add pineapple, rum, bouillon cube and food coloring. Simmer covered for 30 minutes or until done. Add cherries and simmer about 10 minutes longer. Serve with hot rice, or packaged seasoned rice. We serve this with a red leaf and bibb lettuce salad with a sweet-sour dressing and rolls.

CHICKEN CASSEROLE

1 small chicken, cut into 4 pieces
2 medium tomatoes, peeled and chopped
4 tablespoons soft type margarine
4 oz. or ¼ lb. smoked ham, chopped
6 small onions, chopped
1 garlic clove, crushed or chopped (optional)
1 wine glass port
1 wine glass brandy
1 tablespoon mustard
white wine to taste
salt and pepper

Put everything into a large casserole, cover and cook slowly till chicken is done, about 45–50 minutes. Remove the cover the last 15–20 minutes to let the top brown.

CHICKEN WITH MADEIRA

2 boned chicken breasts
2 tablespoons soft type margarine
½ teaspoon dry mustard
2 tablespoons tomato sauce
2 tablespoons chicken broth
salt and pepper to taste
1 small glass dry white wine
Madeira wine

Season the chicken breasts with salt and sauté in the melted margarine. In a separate pan melt a little margarine and add the mustard, tomato sauce, chicken broth and, after mixing thoroughly, add the sauce from the sautéed chicken. Salt and pepper according to desired taste. Add the small glass of dry white wine. Simmer gently till chicken is tender, about 30 minutes. Before serving add a small amount of Madeira.

SOLE IN PARSLEY SAUCE

1 16 oz. package frozen sole fillets, thawed
1 package vegetable bouillon
½ cup water
½ cup chopped carrot
¼ cup chopped celery salt and pepper

3 tablespoons flour
¾ cup skimmed milk or re-liquified non-fat dry milk
1 tablespoon parsley flakes
⅛ teaspoon marjoram, optional

In medium saucepan over medium heat, dissolve bouillon in ½ cup water; add carrot and celery; simmer 10 minutes. Drain vegetables, reserving liquid for sauce. Sprinkle fillets with salt and pepper. Place 2 tablespoons vegetable mixture down center of each fillet. Roll up and secure with toothpick. In same saucepan, stir reserved liquid with flour until smooth; stir in remaining ingredients. Cook over medium heat just until boiling; reduce heat to low. Add fish; cover, simmer, for 15 minutes or until fish flakes. Makes 4 servings.

FISH WITH WINE AND TOMATOES

2 lbs. white fish fillets
2 medium onions, finely chopped
chopped parsley
1 garlic clove, minced
1 tablespoon safflower oil

2 tablespoons soft type margarine
1 cup white wine
2 peeled tomatoes
2 tablespoons tomato juice juice of 1 lemon

Place in a baking dish half the oil and some of the sliced onion and chopped parsley. Place the whole fish on top, then pour over it the lemon and tomato juice, minced garlic, rest of the oil, onion, margarine and wine, tomatoes and other seasonings. Cover and bake in a 350 degree oven for about 30 minutes.

SALMON STEAKS

Make marinade sauce of:

½ cup unsaturated oil	½ teaspoon dry mustard
¼ cup snipped parsley	¼ teaspoon salt
¼ cup lemon juice	dash pepper
2 tablespoons grated onion	

Place 6 fresh salmon steaks in shallow dish. Pour on marinade sauce. Let stand at room temperature for 2 hours, turning occasionally. Drain, reserving marinade. Sauté steaks in small amount of melted soft type margarine, till slightly brown. Baste with marinade. Place in 350 degree oven for about 30 minutes, basting occasionally with sauce.

COD IN WHITE WINE

Place cod fillets in baking dish. Sprinkle with paprika, salt and pepper to taste. Add about ¼ cup white wine. Cover and bake in 350 degree oven about 40 minutes. Serve with lemon slices.

LEG OF LAMB WITH MINT SAUCE

Trim the leg of lamb of excess fat, do not remove the parchment-like covering. Mix salt, finely ground pepper, dried crushed rosemary and rub the mixture firmly into the lamb. Place leg, fat side up, in shallow roasting pan and roast uncovered in oven for 20 minutes (500 degrees). Reduce heat to 375 degrees and roast for another 40–60 minutes or until lamb is cooked to your taste. Serve when done with mint sauce:

¼ cup water
1 tablespoon sugar

¼ cup finely chopped fresh mint leaves
½ cup malt vinegar

Make the mint sauce in advance. Combine water and sugar and bring to boil over high heat, stirring until sugar is dissolved. Remove from heat and stir in mint leaves and vinegar. Set aside at room temperature for 2–3 hours.

STUFFED PORK CHOPS

1 cup soft bread crumbs
½ cup chopped celery
2 tablespoons chopped parsley
3 tablespoons chopped onions
1 tablespoon safflower oil

1 cup cranberry sauce
1 teaspoon salt
pepper
6 lean pork chops, 1 inch thick
2 tablespoons soft margarine
flour

Combine crumbs, celery, parsley, onions, cranberry sauce, and oil. Add salt and pepper. Cut pocket in trimmed pork chops and stuff; sprinkle with salt and pepper and dredge with flour. Brown lightly in margarine, then bake uncovered in 350 degree oven till tender. Serves 6.

WILD DUCK A L'ORANGE

Skin the duck, remove breast bone and divide the breast in two pieces. Clean thoroughly and wipe the meat with toweling. Sauté the breast pieces and legs in margarine, salt to taste and sprinkle with lemon, pepper and crushed marjoram seasoning. Place in baking dish and pour ½ cup orange juice for the liquid. Add more juice if more than 1 bird is being served. Cover and bake for 2½ hours at 350 degrees. You may uncover the last 20 minutes if desired. Serve with orange sauce:

1 small can orange juice, frozen, concentrate plus
1 cup water

½ cup sugar plus 1 tablespoon cornstarch
dash salt, nutmeg and cinnamon
2 tablespoons margarine

Mix thoroughly and simmer on low heat till thickened.

PORK, ORIENTAL STYLE

1 lb. pork cutlet, trimmed of the fat
5 tablespoons soy sauce
1 teaspoon sugar

1 green onion
1 clove garlic
¼ teaspoon chopped ginger

Cut pork into thin pieces and brown in pan. Remove from pan and let stand in mixture of soysauce, sugar, garlic, onion and ginger for 10 minutes. Cook together until pork is tender. Serve with rice and green vegetable.

BEEF WITH MUSHROOMS

1 lb. round steak, trimmed of the fat
½ cup chopped onion
1 cup mushrooms
¼ cup soy sauce

½ cup milk, skim, soured with the addition of ½ tablespoon of vinegar

Cut beef into thin strips and soak in soy sauce. Sauté onions and mushrooms in soft margarine for 2 minutes. Remove from pan and brown meat strips in the margarine. Add onions and mushrooms and let simmer until meat is tender. Add the soured milk just before serving.

VEAL OR BEEF TOMATO

½ lb. of top round steak or veal steak
2 tablespoons cornstarch
1 tablespoon soy sauce
1 tablespoon brandy
2 tablespoons safflower oil
¼ cup chopped onion
⅓ cup sliced celery
¾ cup green pepper cut into 1 inch squares

2 whole tomatoes, peeled, cut into segments
¼ cup sliced water chestnuts
1 cup chicken broth or soup stock, heated
2 tablespoons catsup
½ teaspoon salt
1 tablespoon cornstarch mixed with 3 tablespoons cold water

Slice the beef or veal about ⅛ inch thick. Mix with cornstarch, soy sauce and brandy. Let stand about 30 minutes while you prepare the rest of the ingredients. Heat pan and add oil; add meat and stir-fry until golden brown. Remove from pan and reserve. Add onion and celery and sauté 10–15 seconds, then add rest of vegetables and stir a few minutes. Add heated broth, cover and let steam about 1 minute. Remove cover and add meat and mix well. Cover again and let steam for another 15–20 seconds. Add seasonings and stir a few times. Thicken slightly with cornstarch mixture. Serves 4. Serve with rice.

STEAK DIANE FOR FOUR

4 eight oz. sirloin steaks
For the sauce per portion:
2½ tablespoons of soft type margarine
1 tablespoon cognac, heated
2 tablespoons sherry

1 tablespoon beef bouillon
1 tablespoon chopped chives
1 teaspoon minced parsley salt and pepper to taste

Trim meat well and pound until very thin. Cream 2 tablespoons margarine with chives and parsley, salt and pepper. Melt remaining margarine in chafing dish or frying pan. Add steaks and brown quickly until just seared. Remove to hot platter. Pour warmed cognac into frying pan and flame. Add sherry, seasoned margarine and bouillon. When blended return steak to pan just long enough to reheat it. Serve at once.

BAKED CHICKEN WITH APRICOTS

1 two lb. broiler fryer, cut into serving pieces
salt and pepper
1 tablespoon of soft type margarine
2 tablespoons molasses

1½ tablespoons lemon juice
1 tablespoon finely chopped onion
½ teaspoon ground ginger
canned apricot halves, drained

Heat oven to 375 degrees. Sprinkle chicken with salt and pepper, then place in a shallow baking dish. Combine the margarine, molasses, lemon juice, onion and ginger. Brush this mixture over the chicken. Bake for 35 minutes, basting occasionally. Add apricot halves, baste and cook about 10–15 minutes longer, until the fruit is heated and the chicken is tender.

TURKEY DIVAN

1 package frozen broccoli spears, cooked

8 slices cooked turkey, white meat
4 slices hot toast

In advance prepare Mornay Sauce, cook broccoli, and cut turkey in thick (¼ inch) slices. Preheat oven to 400 degrees. Place 4 slices toast on a 12 x 9 inch dish. Next place a layer of cooked turkey slices. Partially cook and lay on top of meat, 1 package frozen broccoli or asparagus, well drained. Cover with Mornay Sauce. Heat in oven until the sauce is browned and bubbling. Serves 4.

Mornay Sauce:

1 **tablespoon soft type margarine**	2 **tablespoons flour**
	1 **cup skim milk**
1 **teaspoon minced or finely sliced onion**	¼ **cup shredded Cheez-ola cheese**

Melt margarine in skillet. Add onion and cook until onion is yellow. Add flour, cook until mixture bubbles. Slowly stir in milk. Cook over low heat until thickened and smooth. Add ¼ cup shredded cheese; cook, stirring until cheese is melted.

CHICKEN CACCIATORE

2½ **to 3 lb. broiler, quartered**	¼ **teaspoon marjoram**
	2 **bay leaves**
1 **cup chopped onion**	1 **garlic clove**
1 **chicken bouillon cube**	2 **medium sized green**
1 **cup boiling water**	**peppers, seeded and**
1 **tablespoon salt**	**sliced**
½ **teaspoon pepper**	1 **lb. can tomatoes**
dash cayenne pepper	8 **oz. can tomato sauce**

Season chicken with salt and pepper. Brown chicken in broiler on both sides. In skillet add onions, garlic, green pepper, bouillon cube and seasoning to 1 cup boiling water. Add remaining ingredients. Cover, add chicken and simmer 1 hour until tender. Remove cover during last half-hour. Serve sauce over chicken.

CHICKEN CHOW MEIN (AMERICAN STYLE)

1 tablespoon margarine, soft type
4 tablespoons minced onion
1½ cups shredded cooked chicken
1 cup diced celery
1½ cup meat stock or water
2 tablespoons soy sauce
1½ tablespoons cornstarch
3 tablespoons cold water
Chow Mein noodles
Sugar substitute, if desired

Brown onion lightly in margarine. Add next 4 ingredients and simmer 15 minutes. Blend the cornstarch and cold water and stir into meat mixture. Cook until slightly thickened and clear. Serve hot on Chow Mein noodles. Serves 4.

BAKED SPICED PORK CHOPS

4 pork chops trimmed of fat
1 teaspoon seasoned salt
1½ cups hot water
1 tablespoon chicken seasoned stock base
¼ teaspoon orange peel
¼ teaspoon thyme
¼ teaspoon cinnamon
¼ teaspoon allspice
⅛ teaspoon black pepper
1 tablespoon instant minced onion

Brown pork chops in heavy frying pan. Season with seasoned salt. Arrange chops in casserole or baking dish. Dissolve chicken base in hot water. Add orange peel. Crush thyme and add to stock along with cinnamon, allspice, pepper, and onions. Pour over chops. Cover and bake in a 300 degree oven for 1½ hours or until tender. Skim off any excess fat.

FISH AND POTATO CASSEROLE

Cook about 2 lbs. fish steaks or fillets in 1 cup simmering water with 1 teaspoon salt just until it flakes when tested with a fork. Cool, drain, and flake fish (discard any skin or bones); add skim milk to the poaching liquid to make 2 cups; set aside. In 2 tablespoons of the soft margarine, sauté 1 large onion (sliced) until soft; set aside.

Put about 1 quart sliced, cooked potatoes in a 2 or 2½ quart casserole. Top with the flaked, cooked fish (you should have about 1 quart fish). Distribute the onions over potatoes.

In the frying pan, melt 2 tablespoons soft type margarine; add 2 tablespoons flour, 1 teaspoon salt, ¼ teaspoon pepper, and ½ teaspoon thyme; cook, stirring, until bubbly. Gradually stir in the 2 cups reserved liquid (use all milk with leftover fish); cook, stirring until thickened, then pour into casserole. Bake, uncovered, in a 350 degree oven until heated through, about 30 minutes. Makes about 6 servings.

SKILLET PINEAPPLE CHICKEN

3 large chicken breasts, boned, skinned, cut in half
1½ teaspoons salt
2 tablespoons margarine
1 tablespoon instant minced onion
1 cup sliced celery
cold water

1 green pepper, cut into strips
1 8 oz. can pineapple tidbits, unsweetened
1½ teaspoon soy sauce
½ teaspoon cinnamon
2 teaspoons cornstarch

Cut each of the chicken breast halves into 10–12 crosswise strips. Sprinkle with salt. In large skillet over high heat, sauté chicken strips in margarine for 3 minutes, stirring constantly. Add onion, celery, and green pepper;

then continue cooking 2 minutes. Add pineapple, soy sauce, cinnamon and ¼ cup cold water; stir, cover and simmer 4 minutes. Blend cornstarch with 2 tablespoons of cold water; stir into skillet. Cook, stirring until thickened. Makes 6 servings.

SHRIMP WITH CURRY SAUCE

Cook chopped onion and green pepper and celery in unsaturated oil till tender. Add cooked shrimp and 1 can of tomatoes and ½ teaspoon of curry powder. If necessary, thicken this mixture with a little cornstarch. Heat thoroughly. Arrange on a platter and surround this mixture with hot cooked rice. Sprinkle with parsley.

LOBSTER GENOVESE

Brown garlic clove in 1 tablespoon of unsaturated oil. Add parsley, 1 can of tomatoes and salt and pepper. Simmer for 10 minutes. Remove the garlic clove. Place cooked lobster in baking dish and pour sauce over it. Bake 350 degrees for 20 minutes.

SALAD DRESSING

NEVER-FAIL MAYONNAISE

Courtesy, Home Service Department of Corn Products Refining Company

½ teaspoon sugar	1 egg white
½ teaspoon dry mustard	1 cup unsaturated oil
¼ teaspoon salt	4 teaspoons vinegar

Combine sugar, mustard, salt in a bowl. Add egg whites, beat well. Continue beating and add oil a little at a time until ½ cup is used. Add 2 teaspoons vinegar, continue beating, adding the remaining oil. Beat in the last 2 teaspoons of vinegar. Store in a covered jar in refrigerator.

OIL AND VINEGAR DRESSING

½ cup unsaturated oil
¼ cup vinegar
   dash of dry mustard

1 teaspoon salt
¼ teaspoon pepper
   garlic powder, if desired

Mix well and chill.

RUSSIAN SALAD DRESSING

1 cup water
1 cup sugar plus the juice
   of 2 lemons. Boil to
   syrup, cook, add:
2 cups unsaturated oil
1 cup catsup

2 tablespoons Worcester-
   shire Sauce
2 tablespoons grated onion
2 teaspoons celery salt
1 teaspoon salt
1 teaspoon paprika

Beat thoroughly. Chill.

POTATO MAYONNAISE

1 very small baked potato
1 teaspoon mustard
1 teaspoon salt

1 teaspoon powdered sugar
2 tablespoons vinegar
¾ cup unsaturated oil

Remove and mash the inside of the potato. Add mustard, salt and powdered sugar; add 1 tablespoon vinegar and rub mixture through a fine sieve. Slowly add the oil and the remaining vinegar.

SESAME SEED DRESSING

⅔ cup safflower oil
⅓ cup vinegar
1 tablespoon toasted
   sesame seed

1 teaspoon celery salt
1 teaspoon dry mustard
½ teaspoon salt

Shake all ingredients in tightly covered jar. Makes about 1 cup dressing.

SUNSHINE SALAD DRESSING

1 teaspoon prepared
    mustard
1 teaspoon celery salt
½ teaspoon salt
¼ teaspoon pepper
½ cup orange juice

½ cup safflower oil
1 tablespoon honey or
    sugar
2 to 3 teaspoons grated
    onion

Shake all ingredients in tightly covered jar. Chill. Serve on vegetable salad. Makes about 1 cup dressing.

SWEET-SOUR DRESSING

1 cup safflower oil
½ cup red wine vinegar
¼ cup honey
1 teaspoon salt

1 teaspoon dry mustard
1 teaspoon poppy seed
1 teaspoon celery seed

Blend all ingredients with rotary beater or shake well in tightly covered jar. Chill. Makes about 1¾ cups dressing.

CURRY DRESSING

1 teaspoon salt
¼ teaspoon curry powder
¼ teaspoon pepper
    dash cayenne pepper
1 tablespoon grated onion

1 tablespoon minced
    parsley
1 tablespoon grated lemon
    peel
2 tablespoons vinegar
⅓ cup safflower oil

Mix all ingredients. Beat or shake thoroughly. Makes about ½ cup dressing.

ZERO SALAD DRESSING

May be used in any amount.

1 cup tomato juice
¼ cup lemon juice or
    vinegar

2 tablespoons finely
    chopped onion
    salt and pepper

Finely chopped parsley, celery, green pepper in amounts desired may be added.

Optional ingredients: horseradish, dry mustard, garlic. Combine ingredients; shake well before using.

AVOCADO DRESSING

½ cup pureed avocado
1 tablespoon lemon juice
2 tablespoons of French dressing made with safflower oil or corn oil

¼ teaspoon salt
2 tablespoons Poly-Perx cream substitute

Add and blend each ingredient one at a time to the pureed avocado. Blend all together. This is nice for a grapefruit and lettuce salad.

CREAMY MAYONNAISE DRESSING

6 tablespoons of mayonnaisse from the recipe on page 92.

3 tablespoons of Poly-Perx cream substitute

Blend together till smooth. This serves 6.

HONEY DRESSING

1 cup safflower oil
⅓ cup honey
⅓ cup lemon juice
1 tablespoon vinegar
1 teaspoon dry mustard
1 teaspoon celery seed
½ teaspoon salt

½ teaspoon paprika
¼ teaspoon pepper
Non-caloric liquid sweetener equivalent to ⅔ cup sugar
1 tablespoon grated onion or onion juice

Beat all ingredients in bowl with rotary beater or shake

well in tightly covered jar. Chill. Shake before serving on fresh fruit salads. Makes about 2 cups.

FRENCH DRESSING

1 can tomato soup	1 teaspoon mustard, dry
½ cup sugar	1 teaspoon salt
½ cup vinegar	1 teaspoon grated onion
½ cup unsaturated oil	dash of pepper

Mix well and chill.

SWEET SALAD DRESSING

¾ cup sugar	1 teaspoon salt
⅓ cup vinegar	1 teaspoon dry mustard

Boil above ingredients one minute. Cool and add with a wooden spoon: 1 cup of unsaturated oil, 1 teaspoon onion juice. Blend until mixture is very stiff. Celery seed may be added. For grapefruit, avocado or any fruit or vegetable salad.

SALADS

MOLDED COTTAGE CHEESE SALAD

4 cups water	¾ cup chopped walnuts
1 cup cottage cheese	2 packages of lime or
4 tablespoons mayonnaise	lemon Jello
4 grapefruits	

Peel and section grapefruit, cover bottom of 10 x 8 x 2 pyrex dish with half of fruit sections. Cover with half of Jello. Let congeal. Mix mayonnaise, cottage cheese thoroughly, add nuts. Spread on top of the Jello. Add remaining grapefruit and Jello. Refrigerate. Serves 10.

AVOCADO-TUNA SALAD

Avocado, half
French Dressing made
with safflower oil or
corn oil
tuna fish
celery

1 tablespoon onion,
chopped
mayonnaise, recipe on
page 92
¼ teaspoon paprika
¼ teaspoon salt
tomatoes, sliced

Cut avocado in half and remove stone. Marinate for a few minutes in the French dressing. Make a tuna salad with celery, onion, paprika, salt, mayonnaise and the French dressing used to marinate the avocado. Place avocado filled with tuna salad on bed of lettuce and border with sliced tomatoes.

RAW FISH SALAD WITH VEGETABLES

1 to 2 pounds of raw white
fish, bass or tuna or
halibut
6 to 7 fresh limes
tomatoes, sliced, wedged
or chopped

carrots, grated
lettuce
salt and pepper
onion, chopped

Cut fish into ½ to 1-inch squares and marinate in the lime juice for 4 to 6 hours before serving. When fish is cured in the lime juice, remove excess liquids and discard. Arrange fish on bed of lettuce, add other ingredients as a garnish or serve as a tossed salad.

CHINESE CHICKEN SALAD

2 cups cooked chicken
meat
¼ cup soy sauce
¼ teaspoon garlic oil or
pinch of garlic
powder
½ teaspoon sugar

¼ teaspoon ground ginger
1 cup diced celery
½ cup chopped almonds
or walnuts
1 cup fresh or canned
pineapple tidbits

Marinate the chicken in a sauce made from all the remaining ingredients. Serve on a lettuce with Creamy Mayonnaise Dressing, page 95 or French Dressing made with safflower oil or corn oil.

PINEAPPLE-CARROT SALAD

1 package lemon jello
1 cup hot water
1 cup pineapple juice from
    canned fruits

1 cup pineapple tidbits
1 cup grated raw carrots

Dissolve the gelatin in hot water and add pineapple juice. Chill until thickened. Fold in pineapple and carrots. Chill until firm. Serve on lettuce leaves. Serves 6.

FRUIT MEDLEY SALAD

1 envelope (1 tablespoon)
    unflavored gelatin
½ cup unsweetened
    orange juice
1¼ cups boiling water
¼ teaspoon salt
1¼ teaspoons liquid
    sweetener

Food coloring, if
    desired
1 medium pear or apple,
    diced
½ cup Tokay grapes, cut
    in half and seeded

In medium mixing bowl, soften gelatin in orange juice. Stir in boiling water, salt, food coloring and liquid sweetener. Chill until slightly thickened but not set. Carefully stir in fruit. Pour into 3- or 4-cup mold or 6 individual molds. Chill until set, about 4 hours. Serves 6.

CUCUMBERS IN VINAIGRETTE

2 large cucumbers, thinly sliced
4 cups salted ice water
2 or 3 fresh green onions, chopped
½ teaspoon salt
¼ teaspoon pepper
1 teaspoon liquid sweetener
½ cup vinegar

In a large mixing bowl, combine cucumbers and salted ice water. Let stand for 30 minutes, then drain. Add the onions. Combine remaining ingredients and mix well. Pour over cucumbers, tossing lightly. Cover. Chill several hours, stirring occasionally. Makes 8 (½ cup) servings.

GARDEN RELISH SALAD

4 cups finely chopped green cabbage
¾ cup finely chopped carrot
1 medium green pepper, finely chopped
½ cup finely chopped onion
¾ cup cider vinegar
⅓ cup sugar
1 tablespoon salt
½ teaspoon mustard seed
½ teaspoon celery seed

In large bowl, combine vegetables. Combine remaining ingredients in a jar and shake well. Pour dressing over vegetables and toss to coat. Refrigerate covered for several hours before serving. Makes 6 cups.

HOT CHICKEN SALAD

2 cups cubed cooked chicken
2 cups thinly sliced celery
½ cup chopped toasted almonds
½ teaspoon salt
2 teaspoons grated onion
1 cup mayonnaise
2 tablespoons lemon juice
½ cup grated cheese
1 cup toasted bread cubes

Mix all the ingredients together, except the cheese and

bread cubes and pile lightly into baking dish. Sprinkle the ½ cup grated cheese and 1 cup toasted bread cubes over top. Bake until bubbly, 10 to 15 minutes in a 450 degree oven. Serves 6. This is a perfect luncheon dish.

COLE SLAW

Soak cabbage in salted water for ½ hour, then drain it. Shred enough to make 3 cups. Combine with 3 tablespoons diced celery, 3 tablespoons diced green pepper and 3 tablespoons diced pimentos. Mix with Mustard Dressing. Refrigerate at least ½ hour before serving.

MUSTARD DRESSING

1 tablespoon prepared mustard

2 tablespoons lemon juice
dash cayenne pepper

⅔ cup non-fat skim milk powder

⅔ cup water

½ teaspoon salt
dash grated pepper

4 teaspoons sugar

3 cups shredded cabbage

Combine and refrigerate all ingredients except cabbage in mixing bowl. When chilled, whip with electric mixer until quite thick. Combine with 3 cups shredded cabbage.

SALAD SUGGESTIONS

1. Molded salads—fruit and vegetables.
2. Garden Greens—served with oil and vinegar dressing.
3. Lettuce, tomato, radishes and chopped ripe olives and anchovies. Tossed with oil and vinegar dressing.
4. 1 can tuna or other fish, flaked and mixed with diced celery, salt and pepper to taste, ⅛ teaspoon thyme, and ¼ cup canned tomatoes. Blend well and serve on lettuce leaf or as a stuffing for a tomato.
5. Place dry curd cottage cheese in food mixer. Add small amount of skim milk. Blend well. Salt and pepper to

taste. Chives or nut meats may be added, if desired. Serve with fruit or vegetable on lettuce leaves.

CAKES

MAYONNAISE CAKE

1 cup dates, cut	½ cup brown sugar
1 teaspoon soda	2 cups sifted cake flour
1 cup boiling water	2 tablespoons cocoa
1 cup mayonnaise	1 cup chopped walnuts
1 cup white sugar	1 teaspoon cinnamon

Cover dates and soda with water and allow to cool. Add mayonnaise and sugar; stir gently; do not beat. Add the flour and cinnamon mixture. Bake at 350 degrees for about 55 minutes in a pan lined with wax-paper.

LADY BALTIMORE CAKE

2¾ cups sifted cake flour	1 teaspoon grated orange peel
1¾ cups sugar	1 teaspoon vanilla
2½ teaspoons baking powder	½ cup milk
1 teaspoon salt	5 egg whites
⅔ cup soft type margarine	Fluffy White Frosting
¾ skim milk	Fruit Filling

. Preheat oven to 350 degrees. Grease and flour two 9 x 1½ inch layer-cake pans. Sift flour, sugar, baking powder and salt into mixing bowl. Add margarine and ¾ cup milk. Beat 2 minutes at medium speed in electric mixer or 300 strokes by hand; scrape bowl frequently. Add orange peel, vanilla, ½ cup milk and the egg whites; beat for 2 minutes. Pour the mixture into prepared pans. Bake 25 to 30 minutes or until cake springs back when lightly touched with fingertip in the center. Cool in pans 15 minutes. Remove from pans. Cool completely on wire racks before filling and frosting.

FLUFFY WHITE FROSTING

¾ cup sugar
¼ cup water
¼ cup light corn syrup

3 egg whites
1 teaspoon vanilla or
   almond extract

Combine sugar, water and corn syrup in small saucepan. Cook over medium heat until sugar is dissolved and mixture begins to boil. Boil, without stirring, until mixture reaches 242 degrees on candy thermometer or until syrup spins a 6-inch thread from tip of spoon. Just before syrup reaches temperature, beat egg whites until stiff but not dry. Pour syrup in thin stream over egg whites, while beating at high speed. Beat until mixture is stiff and glossy and holds shape. Beat in flavoring. Set aside.

FRUIT FILLING

¼ cup cut-up dried figs
½ cup raisins, chopped
½ cup chopped walnuts

2 tablespoons chopped
   maraschino cherries
1 teaspoon grated orange
   peel

Mix all ingredients. Stir in one-third Fluffy Frosting. Spread between two cake layers. Frost cake with remaining frosting.

WHITE CAKE

2 cups cake flour
2 teaspoons baking
   powder
½ cup soft type margarine
1 cup sugar

⅔ cup skim milk (set in
   warm water)
1 teaspoon vanilla
3 egg whites (4, if small)

Sift flour, measure and add baking powder and sift 3 times. Cream margarine and add sugar gradually. Cream until light and fluffy, add a little flour and milk, one at a time, add vanilla. Beat egg whites, not too dry, fold in, bake in oven 375 degrees for 25 to 30 minutes.

PINEAPPLE FILLING

1 small can pineapple and juice   ½ cup sugar (or more to taste)
3 tablespoons flour

Mix all ingredients in saucepan. Cook about 15 minutes. Frost with boiled frosting.

7-MINUTE ICING

1½ cups sugar   2 egg whites
5 tablespoons water   ⅛ teaspoon cream of tartar

Put all ingredients in upper part of a double boiler and beat over boiling water for from 5 to 7 minutes. Remove and beat until thick.

ICE WATER CAKE

1½ cups sugar   1 cup ice water
½ cup soft margarine   2¼ cups flour
5 egg whites   2 teaspoons baking powder
1 teaspoon vanilla
½ teaspoon almond extract   1 teaspoon salt

Cream margarine and sugar, sift the dry ingredients and add to first mixture alternately with the ice water. Add the vanilla and almond extract. Beat well. Beat the egg whites and fold into the cake batter. Bake 45 minutes at 350 degrees.

BONNIE CAKE

⅔ cup soft type margarine	2¾ cups all-purpose flour
1¾ cups sugar	2½ teaspoons baking powder
3 tablespoons Chono	1 teaspoon salt
⅓ cup water	1⅓ cup skim milk
1½ teaspoons vanilla	

Preheat oven to 350 degrees. Grease and flour baking pan, 13 x 9 x 2 inches or two 8-inch round layer pans. In large mixer bowl, mix margarine, sugar, Chono, water and vanilla until fluffy. Beat 5 minutes on high speed, scraping bowl occasionally. Blend flour, baking powder and salt. Mix in alternately with milk. Batter will be thick. Pour into pan(s). Bake oblong 40 to 50 minutes, layers 30 to 40 minutes, or until wooden pick inserted in center comes out clean. Cool. 24 servings.

BUTTERCUP CAKE

2¼ cups cake flour	½ cup soft type margarine
1½ cups sugar	1 cup buttermilk
1½ teaspoons baking powder	1½ teaspoons vanilla
1 teaspoon salt	3 tablespoons Chono
½ teaspoon soda	⅓ cup water

Preheat oven to 350 degrees. Grease and flour baking pan, 13 x 9 x 2 inches, or two 8-inch round layer pans. Measure all ingredients into large mixer bowl. Mix ½ minute on low speed, scraping bowl constantly. Beat 3 minutes on high speed, scraping bowl occasionally. Pour into pan(s). Bake oblong 35 to 45 minutes, layers 30 to 40 minutes or until wooden pick inserted in center comes out clean. Cool. 24 servings.

GINGERBREAD

2¼ cups Gold Medal
      Flour
  1 teaspoon soda
  1 teaspoon ginger
  1 teaspoon cinnamon
  ½ teaspoon salt
      Low-calorie Orange
      Whipped Topping
      or Low-calorie
      Lemon Sauce

½ cup safflower oil
1 cup dark molasses
1 cup boiling water
1 egg white
2 tablespoons sugar

Preheat oven to 325 degrees. Lightly oil and flour square pan, 9 x 9 x 2 inches. Stir together all dry ingredients except sugar in large bowl. Blend oil, molasses and water. Beat egg white to soft peak stage, gradually adding the sugar. Add oil mixture to the dry ingredients; beat until smooth. Gently fold egg white into batter. Pour into prepared pan. Bake 45 to 50 minutes. Cut and serve warm with topping or sauce. 12 servings.

OLD-FASHIONED GINGERBREAD

2¼ cups Gold Medal
      Flour
  1 teaspoon soda
  1 teaspoon ginger
  1 teaspoon cinnamon
  ½ teaspoon salt
      Low-calorie Orange
      Whipped Topping
      or Low-calorie
      Lemon Sauce

½ cup safflower oil
1 cup dark molasses
1 cup boiling water
1 egg white
2 tablespoons sugar

Preheat oven to 325 degrees. Lightly oil and flour square pan, 9 x 9 x 2 inches. Stir together all dry ingredients except sugar in large bowl. Blend oil, molasses and water. Beat egg white to soft peak stage, gradually adding the sugar. Add the oil mixture to the dry ingredients; beat until smooth. Gently fold egg white into batter. Pour into prepared pan. Bake 45 to 50 minutes. Cut and serve warm with topping or sauce. Twelve servings.

CINNAMON COFFEE CAKE

½ cup brown sugar (packed)	½ cup granulated sugar
½ cup chopped walnuts	2½ teaspoons baking powder
2 tablespoons flour	½ teaspoon salt
2 teaspoons cinnamon	1 egg white
2 tablespoons safflower oil	¼ cup safflower oil
1½ cups Gold Medal Flour	¾ cup skim milk

Preheat oven to 375 degrees. Lightly oil square pan, 8 x 8 x 2 inches. Mix brown sugar, nuts, 2 tablespoons flour, the cinnamon and 2 tablespoons oil; set aside for topping. Stir together 1½ cups flour, the granulated sugar, baking powder and salt. Add egg white, ¼ cup oil and the milk; stir until flour is moistened. Spread half of batter in prepared pan. Sprinkle with half of topping mixture. Spread remaining batter over topping; sprinkle with remaining topping. Bake 30 to 35 minutes. Nine servings.

CHERRY ANGEL FOOD CAKE

1 cup sifted cake flour	¼ cup maraschino cherry juice
1 cup egg whites, plus 1 egg white	1 small bottle maraschino cherries, diced
¼ teaspoon salt	1 tap almond flavoring
1 teaspoon cream of tartar	
1¼ cup sifted granulated sugar	

Beat egg whites until frothy, add salt and cream of tartar. Continue beating until stiff enough to hold up in peaks. Fold in ½ of the sugar, 2 tablespoons at a time. Add flavoring. Fold in small amount at a time; cake flour is sifted once before measuring, sifted 3 times with the rest of the sugar. Add cherries and pour into an ungreased 10-inch angel food pan. Sprinkle top with sugar and bake about 70 minutes at 225 degrees. Invert pan until cake is entirely cold.

POPPY SEED WHITE CAKE

2¾ cups sifted cake flour	4 tablespoons unsaturated oil
¾ teaspoon salt	
3½ teaspoons baking powder	1 teaspoon vanilla
1½ cups sugar	½ cup poppy seeds (soaked in water overnight)
1 cup skim milk	
6 egg whites, stiffly beaten	

Sift dry ingredients together. Add milk. To beaten egg whites add the oil; fold this into the first mixture. Finally add poppy seeds and vanilla. Bake at 375 degrees for about 40 minutes in a wax-paper lined cake pan.

EGGLESS FRUIT CAKE

1 cup buckwheat flour	½ teaspoon cinnamon
2 teaspoons baking powder	¼ cup sugar
¼ teaspoon salt	½ cup molasses
¼ teaspoon allspice	⅓ cup skim milk
¼ teaspoon clove	3 tablespoons coffee
¼ teaspoon mace	½ cup raisins, cut
¼ teaspoon nutmeg	1 cup diced fruit (dry)
	½ cup chopped nuts

Mix and sift dry ingredients. Add fruit and nuts. Mix molasses, milk and coffee and add to the first mixture. Blend thoroughly; pour into a wax-paper lined bread pan and bake at 350 degrees for about 35 minutes.

HAWAIIAN CAKE

2 cups cake flour, sifted
1½ cups sugar
2½ teaspoons baking powder
¼ teaspoon salt
¼ cup water
6 tablespoons unsaturated oil

1 cup crushed pineapple with juice
1 teaspoon vanilla or almond extract
3 egg whites, beaten

Mix the dry ingredients. Mix water, oil, fruit and flavoring. Blend into the dry ingredients. Fold in stiffly beaten egg whites. Pour into a wax-paper lined cake pan and bake at 350 degrees for about 30 minutes.

COCOA CAKE

1 cup sugar
1½ cups flour, sifted
¼ cup cocoa
1 teaspoon soda
¼ teaspoon salt

½ cup sour skim milk
2 egg whites, beaten
¼ cup unsaturated oil
¼ cup boiling water
½ teaspoon vanilla

Sift together the dry ingredients. Add the sour skim milk and blend well. Pour the oil on to the beaten egg whites and then fold into the first mixture. Finally add the boiling water and vanilla. Pour into wax-paper lined cake pan. Bake 325 degrees for 25 minutes. For variety, add ½ cup chopped nuts. Frost and serve.

FROSTINGS AND TOPPINGS

FLUFFY APRICOT SAUCE

Mix ¼ cup hot water with 2 tablespoons of apricot puree. Place over hot water. Add ¼ pound of marshmallow, stir until melted. Serve on Angel Food Cake.

FRESH STRAWBERRY ICING

1 cup fresh strawberries
1 egg white
1 cup powdered sugar

Put into a large bowl and beat. This is excellent with Angel Food cake.

HARVEST MOON FROSTING

2 egg whites, beaten
1 cup brown sugar, firmly packed
dash of salt
¼ cup water
1 teaspoon vanilla
¾ cup walnuts, chopped

Put egg whites, sugar, salt and water in top of double boiler. Beat with egg beater until thoroughly mixed. Place over rapidly boiling water, beating constantly with egg beater, and cook 7 minutes or until frosting will stand in peaks. Remove from heat, add vanilla, and beat until thick enough to spread. Decorate with nuts.

MOCHA ICING

1 tablespoon of unsaturated oil
2 tablespoons of cocoa, added gradually
pinch of salt
2 tablespoons of strong hot coffee
1 cup powdered sugar

Beat until thick and smooth.

WHITE ICING

3 cups confectioner's
   sugar
4 tablespoons hot water

1 egg white, unbeaten
   dash of salt
1 teaspoon of vanilla

Combine sugar and hot water. Add egg white. Beat until smooth.

APPLE SNOW FROSTING

3 tablespoons of grated apple and a little lemon juice. Cover with 1 cup sugar (to prevent its turning dark). Beat the white of 1 egg, then add apple and sugar, and beat until stiff.

HONEY FROSTING

½ cup honey
1 large tablespoon marsh-
   mallow cream

1 egg white
   few drops of lemon
   extract

Boil honey until it forms a firm ball when tried in cold water. Add marshmallow cream; pour slowly over the beaten white of egg and beat until cold. Add lemon flavoring and spread on cake. If a stiffer frosting is wanted, stir over hot water and fold gently over and over for 2 minutes.

FOAMING PUDDING SAUCE

2 egg whites
1 cup confectioner's sugar

½ cup hot skim milk
1 teaspoon vanilla

Beat egg whites until stiff; add sugar gradually and continue beating; add milk and vanilla.

COCOA FROSTING

5¼ tablespoons cocoa	3 tablespoons skim milk,
3 tablespoons unsatu-	heated
rated oil	1½ cups powdered sugar
1 teaspoon vanilla	pinch of salt

Combine all ingredients and stir until smooth. If a thicker consistency is desired, add more powdered sugar.

LOW-CALORIE TOPPINGS

WHIPPED TOPPING

½ cup non-fat dry milk	1 tablespoon lemon juice
½ cup iced water	½ teaspoon vanilla
1 egg white	¼ cup sugar

In small mixer bowl whip non-fat dry milk, iced water and egg white for 3 minutes on high speed. Add lemon juice and whip 1 minute longer on high speed. Gradually add vanilla and sugar; blend on low speed for 1 minute. Serve immediately. Makes 4 cups. Freeze any unused portion for a dessert. Seven calories per tablespoon.

ORANGE WHIPPED TOPPING

½ cup non-fat dry milk	2 tablespoons lemon juice
½ cup chilled orange juice	¼ cup sugar
1 egg white	

In small mixer bowl whip dry milk, orange juice and egg white on high speed 3 minutes or until soft peaks form. Add lemon juice; beat on high speed 1 minute longer. Gradually add sugar; blend on low speed 1 minute. Serve immediately. Makes 3½ cups.

DESSERTS

PLUM PUDDING—UNCOOKED

Dissolve 1 package of lemon Jello in 2 cups of boiling water.

1 cup grapenuts
1 cup soaked dates, cut
1 cup chopped walnuts
    pinch of salt

1 cup chopped cooked
    prunes
¼ teaspoon cloves
½ teaspoon cinnamon

Add above ingredients to the Jello mixture and mix well. Pour into molds and chill. Serve with Orange Sauce or Benedictine Sauce.

ORANGE SAUCE

1½ tablespoons cornstarch
⅓ cup sugar
1 tablespoon grated
    orange rind

1 cup orange juice
½ cup water
1 tablespoon lemon juice

Combine cornstarch, sugar and orange rind. Stir in orange juice and water. Bring to a boil, stirring constantly; boil until clear. Add lemon juice. Serve cold. Makes about 1½ cups.

BENEDICTINE SAUCE

⅓ cup sugar
1 tablespoon cornstarch

¾ cup water
½ cup Benedictine

Combine sugar and cornstarch in a saucepan. Stir in cold water. Cook over low heat, stirring constantly, until sauce is clear. Pour into a bowl and add the Benedictine just before serving. Other liqueurs may be substituted for the Benedictine.

BROWNIES

4 egg whites, stiffly beaten
1¼ cups brown sugar
½ cup flour
1 teaspoon vanilla

3½ tablespoons cocoa
1 tablespoon unsaturated oil
1 cup chopped walnuts

Mix all the ingredients thoroughly. Bake in 9-inch greased pan for about 20 minutes at 325 degrees. Cool. Cut into serving pieces. Dust with powdered sugar.

DATE DELIGHT

12 dates, cut fine
3 egg whites, stiffly beaten
1 cup chopped walnuts

1 cup sugar
12 crushed vanilla wafers
½ teaspoon almond extract

Mix together. Put into 9-inch greased pie pan. Bake at 350 degrees for 30 minutes. Cut. Serve with sherbet.

JELLO SHERBET

Dissolve 2 packages of strawberry or raspberry Jello as directed on box, using juice with the water. When it starts to congeal, stir 1 package of thawed frozen berries (or canned), ¼ cup chopped walnuts and 1 quart of sherbet. Pour into sherbet dishes; chill and serve.

CRANBERRY ICE

Cook 1 package cranberries in 2 cups of water until berries pop. Put through sieve. While hot, add ¾ cup of sugar and juice of 1 orange, plus grated peel. Freeze in tray.

PRUNE SOUFFLE

1 cup prune pulp
½ cup sugar
1 tablespoon lemon juice
1 teaspoon grated lemon
   rind

5 egg whites
¼ teaspoon cream of
   tartar
¼ teaspoon salt

To the prune pulp, add half the sugar. Heat to boiling point and add lemon juice and rind. Beat egg whites until frothy; sprinkle with cream of tartar and salt and beat until stiff but not dry. Gradually beat in remaining sugar. Gently fold egg whites into prune pulp. Turn into a 1½ quart baking dish which has been greased and sprinkled with an even coat of granulated sugar. Bake 325 degree oven for 50–60 minutes. Serve hot or cold. Makes 6 servings.

RITZ DELIGHT

20 Ritz crackers, rolled
   fine
½ cup chopped nuts
1 cup sugar
1 teaspoon baking
   powder

1 teaspoon of salt
3 stiffly beaten egg
   whites
1 teaspoon vanilla

Mix crackers, nuts, sugar, baking powder and salt. Add vanilla to the beaten whites. Fold into the dry ingredients. Bake in greased 9-inch pan at 350 degree oven for 20 minutes. When cool cut for cookies of desired size. Top with fruit. Soda crackers may be used in place of Ritz crackers. ¾ cup of finely chopped dates may be also added for variety.

APPLE BETTY

2 tablespoons sugar
¼ teaspoon cinnamon
½ teaspoon grated
   orange rind
1 cup soft bread crumbs
1½ tablespoons unsatu-
   rated oil

2 large apples, peeled and
   sliced
3 tablespoons water
1 tablespoon orange juice

Mix together 1 tablespoon of sugar, cinnamon, grated orange rind and bread crumbs. Add oil and toss until well mixed. Place ⅓ of this mixture in the bottom of a small casserole. Place half the apple slices on top of crumbs. Add another layer using a third of crumbs, then remaining apples. Mix water, orange juice and remaining sugar; pour over apples; top with crumbs. Cover and bake in 375 degree oven for 20 minutes; remove cover and bake 15 minutes longer or until apples are tender.

ANGEL PIE

4 egg whites
1 cup sugar

¼ teaspoon cream of
   tartar
dash of salt

Beat egg whites with salt until they form at least five peaks on the beater. Then slowly add sugar and cream of tartar. Put in a well-greased pan and bake at 300 degrees for about an hour. When cool, top with fresh fruits and sherbet and finely chopped nuts.

GREEN GAGE PLUM ICE

½ cup sugar
1 cup hot water
1 pint Green Gage
   Plums

1 cup orange juice
2 tablespoons lemon
   juice

Dissolve sugar in hot water; bring to boiling point, then cool. Puree the plums to make pulp. Combine the pulp, orange and lemon juice. Add sugar syrup and juice of plums. Freeze. Makes 1 quart.

APPLE-NUT PUDDING

¾ cup sugar
2 egg whites
½ cup flour
2 finely chopped peeled apples
1 teaspoon baking powder
½ cup nuts, chopped
1 teaspoon almond extract

Beat egg whites and add sugar. Beat thoroughly. Add sifted dry ingredients and then remaining ingredients. Pour into greased pie pan or square pan. Bake in 350 degree oven for 35 minutes. Cool before cutting.

SPICY FRUIT PUDDING

1 package lemon or orange gelatin
2 tablespoons lemon juice
1 tart apple, diced
1 cup ready-to-eat wheat cereal
1 cup raisins, ground
6 pitted dates, diced
½ teaspoon ground cinnamon
dash of ground ginger
¼ teaspoon salt
½ cup nuts, chopped

Make and chill gelatin mixture until jelly-like. Add remaining ingredients. Mold. Chill several hours before serving.

COCOA PUDDING

4 tablespoons cornstarch
4 tablespoons sugar
1 teaspoon vanilla
3 tablespoons cocoa
2 cups skim milk
½ cup chopped nuts
2 egg whites

Scald milk in double boiler. Mix cornstarch, sugar and cocoa; wet to a paste with a little cold water, then stir into the scalded milk and continue to stir until thick. Continue cooking for 30 minutes, stirring frequently. Beat egg whites until stiff and fold into the cornstarch mixture. Add vanilla and nuts. Let cool.

BAKED PEACHES

8 peaches, fresh, with skins on. Simmer 1½ cups brown sugar with 1½ cups water. Mix 3 tablespoons of cornstarch with a little cold water; add to the hot mixture and pour over the peaches. Bake 15–20 minutes at 350 degrees.

APPLE CHARLOTTE

3 cups sweetened apple-
   sauce
1 tablespoon gelatin

¼ cup cold water
½ teaspoon cinnamon
2 egg whites

Choose tart-flavored apples, adding a little lemon juice, if necessary, to bring out the flavor. Soak gelatin in cold water 5 minutes. Melt in a little of the hot applesauce; add cinnamon and the rest of applesauce. Chill until it begins to congeal. Beat egg whites stiff and add to the applesauce. Pour into mold or serving dishes.

DATE AND NUT TORTE

1 cup sugar
3 egg whites, stiffly beaten
6 graham crackers

1 cup nuts, chopped
½ lb. dates, chopped
1 teaspoon vanilla

Add the sugar gradually to the stiffly beaten egg whites. Crush crackers fine; combine with nuts, dates, flavoring and add to egg whites. Pour into greased pie plate. Bake in 350 degree oven for 30 minutes. Serve.

REBECCA PUDDING

4 cups scalded skim milk	**½ cup cold skim milk**
½ cup cornstarch	**1 teaspoon vanilla**
¼ cup sugar	**3 egg whites, stiffly beaten**
¼ teaspoon salt	

Mix cornstarch, sugar and salt in cold milk. Add to scalded milk, stirring constantly until thick, afterwards occasionally; cook 15 minutes. Add flavoring and whites of eggs beaten stiff. Mold and chill.

RASPBERRY WHIP

1½ cups raspberries	**1 egg white, stiffly beaten**
1 cup powdered sugar	

Put ingredients in bowl and beat until stiff enough to hold in shape. Pile lightly on dish. Chill. Strawberry whip may be prepared the same way.

PIE CRUST

1 cup sifted flour	**¼ cup unsaturated oil**
½ teaspoon salt	**2½ tablespoons ice water**

Sift flour and salt together. Combine oil and water. Beat until creamy. Pour all at once over the flour mixture. Mix with fork. Form into ball and roll out dough between two pieces of wax-paper. Remove top sheep of paper; invert dough over pie pan and fold edge and flute. Prick surface of crust for a baked shell and place in 475 degree oven for 10–12 minutes.

AMBROSIA CHIFFON PIE

1 package orange gelatin
½ cup hot water
1 cup orange juice
2 egg whites, stiffly beaten

1 cup powdered sugar
1 cup halved seeded Tokay
grapes
1 baked pie shell

Dissolve gelatin in hot water. Add orange juice. Chill until slightly thick; beat until light. Fold in the beaten egg whites and sugar. Chill until almost firm; add grapes and pour into pie shell. Garnish with sections of oranges.

CRACKER PIE

3 egg whites
1 cup sugar
1 teaspoon baking powder
½ teaspoon vanilla

¾ cup chopped walnuts
1 cup Ritz cracker crumbs
vanilla ice milk

Beat egg whites until stiff. Add sugar, baking powder and vanilla. Mix well. Fold in nuts. Add cracker crumbs. Pour into well-greased 8-inch pie plate. Bake 30 minutes at 350 degrees. Let cool. Cut in wedges and top with ice milk.

CHERRY FRAPPÉ

1 envelope low calorie
cherry flavor gelatin
½ cup boiling water
5 maraschino cherries

1 tablespoon maraschino
cherry syrup
2½ cups crushed ice

Place gelatin and boiling water in blender. Blend until gelatin is dissolved. Add cherries and syrup and continue to blend until mixture is fluffy. Add crushed ice and blend until mixture is the consistency of ice cream, about 3–4 minutes. Serve at once in a cup or glass. Or pour into 6-ounce paper cups and freeze for future use. Remove frozen frappés from freezer 15 minutes before serving. Garnish with mint, if desired.

BAKED ALASKA

Remove center from an Angel Food cake. Leave bottom of cake for liner. Beat 6 egg whites to peak. Add ¼ cup of granulated sugar to egg whites. Cover bottom layer with ½ gallon of your favorite ice milk. Cover cake and ice milk with egg whites. Bake in preheated 400 degree oven for 8–10 minutes (until slightly brown). Serve immediately or place in freezer.

STRAWBERRY SOUFFLÉ

1 cup sugar	5 egg whites stiffly beaten
4 tablespoons water	2 teaspoons Kirsch (with
⅔ cup fruit purée	pineapple, use rum)

Bring sugar and water to a boil until hard ball is formed when dropped in cold water. Add purée and cook gently for a few minutes. While still hot add Kirsch and pour it in a trickle on the egg whites, folding in gently. Pour into a soufflé dish, buttered and sprinkled with sugar, and cook in a moderate, preheated oven, 375 degrees about 30 minutes. Yields 4 servings.

BANANA SOUFFLÉ

4 bananas	4 egg whites, beaten stiffly
1 tablespoon sugar	sugar
1 wine glass port	vanilla extract

Place finely sliced bananas in baking dish with the 1 tablespoon sugar sprinkled on top and the port poured over the surface. Add the sugar and vanilla extract according to taste to the stiffly beaten egg whites. Top the bananas with this meringue. Bake 350 degree oven for about 20 minutes.

STRAWBERRY SHORTCAKE

Shortcake Biscuit:

1 cup flour	**¾ teaspoon salt**
2 teaspoons baking powder	**⅓ stick corn oil margarine**
4 teaspoons sugar	**⅜ cup skim milk**

Sift flour, sugar, salt, and baking powder together. Soften margarine but do not melt. Cut into flour mixture with pastry blender or fork to rice-sized lumps. Add milk to flour mixture to make a fairly soft dough. Knead lightly and turn out on floured bread board or pastry cloth. Pat and roll to ⅛-inch thickness, cut into 16 3-inch rounds. Bake at 425 degrees until lightly browned. Serve with crushed strawberries.

MELON PARFAITS

2⅔ cups Quaker Life cereal	**1 cup small honeydew melon balls**
1 cup small cantaloupe balls	

In tall glasses or cereal bowls alternate layers of Quaker Life cereal, cantaloupe and honeydew melon. Garnish each serving with a maraschino cherry. Serve with skim milk. Makes 4 servings.

SPRING PARFAIT

1¼ ounce envelope low calorie pudding mix	**2 cups skimmed milk**
	2 pints strawberries

Early in the day, prepare pudding as label directs. Cover surface with waxed paper.

Before serving, beat the prepared pudding with a spoon until light and fluffy (a minute or two). Reserve 4 strawberries for garnish. Slice remaining berries crosswise. In

4 parfait glasses alternate layers of pudding and strawberries. Garnish with berries. Serves 4.

BANANA CRISP

5 medium sized bananas	¼ cup soft margarine
¼ teaspoon salt	⅓ cup brown sugar
½ cup vanilla wafer crumbs	¼ teaspoon cinnamon

Slice bananas crosswise into ½-inch slices and arrange in greased casserole. Sprinkle them with salt. Combine vanilla crumbs with margarine using pastry blender, finger tips or a fork. Add sugar and cinnamon, blend. Sprinkle evenly over bananas. Bake at 350 degrees for 20 minutes or until top is browned. Can be served with ice milk.

STRAWBERRY SUPREME

1½ cups finely crushed vanilla wafers	4 egg whites
2 tablespoons sugar	½ cup sugar
4 tablespoons soft type margarine melted	1 pint fresh strawberries, hulled and sliced

Combine crumbs, the sugar (2 tablespoons) and melted margarine. Press into 9 x 9-inch baking dish. In a large mixing bowl beat egg whites till soft peaks form. Gradually add the ½-cup sugar, beating till stiff peaks form. Spread meringue over crumbs. Bake in 350 degree oven for 15–17 minutes. Cool. Spread strawberries over the top. Chill. Serves 8.

APPLE DESSERT

6 apples	½ cup brown sugar
2 tablespoons sugar	½ cup butter
⅛ teaspoon salt	1 cup finely chopped or shaved nuts
¼ teaspoon cinnamon	

Spread bottom and sides of oblong cake pan, 8 x 12 inches, generously with soft margarine. Peel apples, cut into 8 equal parts and place in parallel rows closely in pan. Mix sugar, salt and cinnamon and sprinkle over apples. Cream brown sugar and margarine; add nuts. Spread over and between apples, then pat to make a smooth surface. Bake for ½ hour in quick oven (450 degrees) or until apples are tender. Serves 6. You could pour some Poly-Perx cream substitute over the dessert.

LEMON SHERBET

2 cups sugar
1 teaspoon lemon extract
juice of 2 lemons

4 cups skim milk
2 egg whites, beaten stiff

Mix sugar, extract and juice. Add milk and egg whites. Pack at once in freezer in finely chopped ice and rock salt and freeze. Serves 8.

BRANDY CREAM

Take 1 quart of good quality vanilla ice milk and place in blender. Add 5 ounces of good quality brandy. Mix thoroughly in the blender. Pour into ice tray and place in the freezer compartment of the refrigerator for several hours. Spoon into dessert glasses. Delicious.

MAPLEY BAKED FRUIT

½ cup Aunt Jemima Syrup
¼ cup lemon juice
1 tablespoon soft type margarine
4 fresh or canned pear halves, pared and cut in half lengthwise

2 bananas, sliced
¼ pound green seedless grapes
4 maraschino cherries

Combine syrup and lemon juice in small saucepan. Bring to boil; reduce heat and simmer 5 minutes. Remove from heat and stir in margarine. Place pears, bananas, grapes and cherries in shallow 1-quart casserole. Pour syrup over and bake in preheated moderate oven (375 degrees) for 15–20 minutes or until thoroughly heated. Makes 4 servings.

VEGETABLES

PEAS AND CELERY

⅓ cup coarsely chopped celery
1 10-ounce package frozen peas
½ teaspoon thyme leaves
¼ teaspoon salt

In covered medium saucepan over medium heat, cook celery with ½ cup water 5 minutes or until tender. Add peas, cover, and cook 8 to 10 minutes. Drain. Sprinkle peas with thyme and salt. Makes 4 servings.

CABBAGE WITH CARAWAY SEEDS

1 medium head cabbage (1½ to 2 pounds)
1 teaspoon salt
1 teaspoon margarine, soft type
½ teaspoon caraway seeds

Cut cabbage in 6 wedges. In large saucepan over medium heat, bring ¼ cup water and salt to a boil; add cabbage. Cook covered 7–11 minutes or until tender. Drain off remaining water; toss cabbage and remaining ingredients. Makes 6 servings.

ASPARAGUS PAR EXCELLENCE

1 onion, peeled, chopped
1 green pepper, seeded,
    chopped
2 teaspoons salt
¼ teaspoon pepper
2 10-ounce packages
    frozen asparagus
    spears

2 teaspoons snipped
    pimento
½ teaspoon tarragon
2 teaspoons parsley

In medium-sized skillet, barely cover the chopped onion, green pepper, salt and pepper with cold water; over high heat bring to boil; then reduce heat to low and simmer 5 minutes. Lay frozen asparagus in skillet over low heat, cover; simmer 10–15 minutes, or until tender. In serving dish arrange asparagus; surround with onion-pepper mixture; sprinkle with pimento, tarragon and parsley. Makes 6 servings.

BAKED EGGPLANT

1 medium sized eggplant,
    pared, cut into ½-
    inch cubes
1 pound can solid pack
    tomatoes
1 small green pepper
½ teaspoon salt

½ teaspoon garlic powder
1 medium sized onion
¼ pound fresh or canned
    mushrooms
½ teaspoon oregano
1 stalk celery

Parboil eggplant in small amount of water for 6 minutes. Drain. Combine other ingredients in a large bowl. Arrange tomato mixture and eggplant in layers beginning and ending with tomato mixture. Bake for 1 hour at 350 degrees. Makes 4 servings.

CURRIED SPINACH

2 10-ounce packages
   frozen chopped
   spinach
1 teaspoon salt
⅛ teaspoon pepper
⅛ teaspoon nutmeg
¼ teaspoon curry powder
2 tablespoons soft type
   margarine

Cook spinach according to package directions; add salt. Meanwhile in small saucepan, melt butter. Remove from heat, stir in pepper, nutmeg, and curry powder. Drain spinach well through fine strainer. Return to original pan, then quickly add margarine mixture and toss. Makes 6 servings.

FLUFFY ACORN SQUASH

2 acorn squash, cut in
   halves
1 tablespoon skimmed or
   reliquified non-fat dry
   milk
½ teaspoon cinnamon
¼ to ½ teaspoon allspice
½ teaspoon salt

Preheat oven to 400 degrees. On large cookie sheet, place squash cut side down; bake 30 minutes or until tender. Remove from oven and cool slightly. With spoon, carefully scoop squash from shells into medium bowl. Reserve 2 shells. Mash squash; beat in remaining ingredients. Refill reserved shells; if desired, sprinkle lightly with cinnamon.

OKRA AND TOMATOES

1 can (1 pound) cut okra
1 can (8 ounces) stewed
   tomatoes
½ teaspoon dried crushed
   basil

Heat okra in its liquid, drain and return to saucepan. Add tomatoes and basil and reheat. Makes 4 servings.

MAPLE SWEET POTATOES

6 medium sized sweet
  potatoes
½ cup maple syrup
1 tablespoon soft type
  margarine

1 teaspoon salt
1 cup apple cider or apple
  juice
½ cup water

Boil potatoes in jackets until nearly done. Peel, slice and put in baking pan. Combine other ingredients in a saucepan and bring to a boil. Pour mixture over potatoes and bake in a slow oven 300 degrees for 1 hour until potatoes are glazed.

BAKED TOMATOES SUPREME

2 large ripe tomatoes
4 drops liquid sweetener
1 tablespoon minced scallion

1 tablespoon minced parsley

Slice tomatoes in half. Place half on large square of double thick foil. Sprinkle with sweetener, minced scallions and parsley. Bring foil up and around tomato half. Seal edge of foil, but leave space at top for steaming. Bake at 350 degrees for 20 minutes. Makes 4 servings.

CARROT MEDLEY

1 pound carrots, thinly
  sliced
1 medium onion, thinly
  sliced

3 large stalks celery, cut in
  1 inch slices

Over medium heat, in salted water, cook carrots, onion and celery until tender, about 15 minutes. Drain. Stir in soft type margarine, if allowed in diet.

CURRIED POTATOES

2 cups cold boiled potato cubes

3 tablespoons onion, chopped

½ cup clear chicken broth

6 tablespoons soft margarine

1½ teaspoons curry powder

1 teaspoon lemon juice

Cook onion in margarine until soft. Add potatoes and cook until all the margarine is absorbed, then add chicken broth, curry powder and lemon juice. Salt and pepper to taste. Cook again until all broth has been absorbed by the potatoes.

CHINESE PEAS

1 pound of Chinese peas

½ cup chopped almonds

½ cup sliced mushrooms

1 tablespoon soft margarine

Remove string from peas leaving them in edible pod. Cook in boiling salted water (1 cup) for 4 minutes. Sauté almonds and mushrooms in margarine for 2 minutes. Add to cooked peas. Let simmer together for 1 minute, then serve.

SWEET-SOUR ZUCCHINI

2 tablespoons of unsaturated oil

4 teaspoons of cornstarch

1 tablespoon sugar

1 tablespoon instant minced onion or fresh chopped onions

2 teaspoons prepared mustard

¾ teaspoon salt

½ teaspoon garlic salt dash pepper

½ cup water

¼ cup vinegar

4 cups bias-sliced zucchini

1 cup bias-sliced celery

2 tomatoes, peeled and quartered

In skillet, stir together first 8 items. Add the water and vinegar. Cook, stirring till mixture thickens and boils. Add zucchini and celery, cook, covered 7–8 minutes or till vegetables are tender but crisp, stirring occasionally. Add tomatoes, cook covered 2–3 minutes more or till heated through. Serves 6.

COOKIES

FRUIT BITES (UNBAKED)

½ cup dates	½ teaspoon grated lemon rind
½ cup dried apricots	
½ cup raisins	½ teaspoon grated orange rind
½ cup walnuts	

Put all ingredients through a medium-coarse food chopper. Mix well. Form into small balls and roll in powdered sugar.

CHINESE-CHEWS

1 cup walnuts	1 egg white
½ cup sugar	1 teaspoon vanilla

Grind nuts with medium-coarse food chopper. Add sugar, vanilla and unbeaten egg whites. Let stand for 30 minutes. Shape into little balls the size of a marble. Roll in granulated sugar. Flatten each one slightly with half pecan. Bake at 300 degree oven for 15 minutes.

OATMEAL COCOA (UNBAKED)

3 cups quick cooking oatmeal	½ cup chopped nuts
	½ cup raisins

Mix 2 cups sugar, ¼ cup cocoa, 3 tablespoons unsaturated oil, ⅔ cups skim milk and 3 teaspoons vanilla. Cook this for 5 minutes. Pour over the oatmeal mixture and drop on waxed paper. Makes about 3 dozen.

WHISKEY BALLS (UNBAKED)

2½ cups Nabisco vanilla
    wafers
½ cup rum
3 tablespoons bourbon
    or brandy

1 cup nuts, ground
1 cup powdered sugar
2 tablespoons cocoa
3 tablespoons Karo syrup

Grind vanilla wafers and nuts. Add dry ingredients and mix well. Then add the rum and bourbon and drip in the Karo. Mix thoroughly and roll into balls. Roll in powdered sugar and store in air-tight container. These improve with age.

CRISP GINGER SNAPS

1 cup sugar
6 tablespoons unsatu-
    rated oil
¼ teaspoon salt
4 tablespoons skim milk
    or molasses

2 egg whites
1 teaspoon cinnamon
½ teaspoon clove
½ teaspoon ginger
2 cups flour, sifted
2 teaspoons soda

Mix the dry ingredients together. Fluff the egg whites; add the oil and skim milk. Blend the two mixtures together. Form dough into small balls the size of a walnut. Dip in sugar. Bake at 350 degrees for about 10 minutes.

PECAN KISSES

Beat 2 egg whites until stiff, gradually add ½ cup sugar. Beat until thick and glossy. Fold in ¼ teaspoon vanilla and ¾ cup chopped nuts. Drop by spoonful on a greased baking sheet. Bake at 250 degrees for about 30 minutes or until delicately brown.

GINGER SNAPS

1 cup soft margarine	2 teaspoons ginger
1 cup molasses	½ teaspoon salt
1 teaspoon soda	2½ cups flour, sifted

Boil margarine and molasses 2 minutes and cool. Add soda, ginger, salt and flour to make a stiff dough. Chill in refrigerator several hours or overnight. Roll very thin. Bake in 375 degree oven for about 8 minutes. About 50 cookies.

ALMOND-DATE COOKIES

¼ teaspoon salt	1½ tablespoons water
½ cup soft margarine	½ tablespoon vanilla
1 cup confectioner's sugar	1 cup chopped almonds
2 cups flour, sifted	halves of pitted dates

Cream salt, margarine, sugar together. Sift flour into mixture. Add water and vanilla. Blend. Add chopped almonds. Wrap a teaspoonful of the batter around a pitted date half. Bake at 325 degrees for about 12 minutes. Cook on ungreased baking sheet. While still warm roll cookies in confectioner's sugar.

CHEWY OATMEAL COOKIES

2 cups quick cooking oats	2 egg whites
1 cup brown sugar (packed)	¼ teaspoon salt
½ cup safflower oil	½ teaspoon almond extract

Heat oven to 325 degrees. Stir together oats, sugar and oil in mixing bowl. Beat egg whites until frothy and add to oat mixture. Stir in salt and almond extract. Drop mixture by teaspoonfuls on lightly oiled baking sheet. Bake about 15 minutes. Cool; remove from baking sheet. Makes about 3 dozen cookies.

STIR-N-DROP SUGAR COOKIES

3 egg whites	¾ cup sugar
⅔ cup safflower oil	2 cups Gold Medal Flour
2 teaspoons vanilla	2 teaspoons baking
1 teaspoon grated lemon	powder
peel	½ teaspoon salt

Heat oven to 400 degrees. Beat egg whites with fork until frothy. Stir in oil, vanilla and peel. Blend in sugar until mixture thickens. Stir together flour, baking powder and salt; blend in. Drop dough by teaspoonfuls about 2 inches apart on ungreased baking sheet. Flatten with oiled bottom of glass dipped in sugar. Bake 8–10 minutes or until a delicate brown. Remove from baking sheet immediately. Makes about 4 dozen 2½-inch cookies.

OATMEAL COOKIES

½ cup soft type margarine	½ teaspoon baking soda
⅔ cup sugar	1 cup all-purpose flour
1 teaspoon vanilla	½ teaspoon salt
1 tablespoon and 1 tea-	¾ cup cold water
spoon "chono" (egg	½ cup raisins
substitute)	1 cup rolled oats
1 teaspoon cinnamon	

Preheat oven to 375 degrees. In large mixer bowl, combine margarine, sugar, vanilla, and Chono. Beat 2 minutes at high speed, scraping bowl occasionally, until well blended. Add flour, cinnamon, salt, soda, and water. Beat at low speed until well combined, about 2 minutes. Stir in rolled oats and raisins. (Dough will be soft.) Drop by teaspoons, 2 inches apart, onto ungreased cookies sheets. Bake at 375 degrees for 12 to 15 minutes, until cookies are set. Store in refrigerator. Makes 42 cookies.

SESAME COOKIES

1 cup soft type margarine	¼ teaspoon salt
¼ cup powdered sugar	⅔ cup sesame seeds
2¼ cup flour	1 teaspoon vanilla

Cream margarine and sugar; sift flour and salt and add to mixture. Then add vanilla and sesame seeds. Mix well. Roll into balls (1 rounded teaspoonful) and flatten. Bake on ungreased cookie sheet in preheated oven 350 degrees for 10 minutes.

Dip cookies in powdered sugar once while hot and again when cool.

OAT SQUARES

1 cup brown sugar	¼ teaspoon salt
⅓ cup soft type margarine	2 cups oatmeal

Mix margarine and sugar in small 8 x 9-inch bake pan. Add salt and oatmeal. When thoroughly mixed, press down firmly and place in oven. Cook at 350 degrees for 30 minutes. Let cool and then cut into squares.

LEMON WAFERS

½ cup flour, sifted	½ teaspoon grated lemon rind
¼ cup margarine, soft type	1 teaspoon lemon juice
¼ cup sifted powdered sugar	2 tablespoons skim milk

Sift flour once, measure, and sift again. Cream margarine thoroughly, add lemon rind and juice and blend. Add flour, alternately with milk, mixing well. Drop ¼ teaspoon on an ungreased baking sheet, placing about 2 inches apart. Bake in 375 degree oven about 5 minutes. Makes about 3 dozen wafers.

MARGUERITES

3 tablespoons water	1 egg white
1/8 teaspoon salt	3/4 cup sugar
1/8 teaspoon cream of tartar	3/4 teaspoon vanilla
or 1 teaspoon light	2 dozen salted soda
corn syrup	crackers

Cook all ingredients except crackers as for Seven-Minute Frosting. Drop a mound of frosting from a teaspoon on each cracker. Bake at 350 degrees about 15 minutes or until delicately brown. Cool on cake rack. These are best served the same day.

JORDAN SPECIALS

3 egg whites	1/2 pound chopped Jordan
1/2 pound powdered sugar	almonds
1 tablespoon cinnamon	rind of 1/2 lemon
	1/4 teaspoon salt

Add salt to egg whites and beat until stiff, but not dry. Gradually beat in powdered sugar, adding a small amount at a time. When nearly all of the powdered sugar is added, fold in remaining sugar with cinnamon and lemon rind. Then add nuts, chopped but not blanched. Dredge a board with flour, then with powdered sugar, and turn the mixture onto the board. Roll out to 1/3 inch in thickness, then cut with a small cookie cutter. Put into shallow, well-greased baking pan and bake at 300 degrees for about 1/2 hour. Spread with a tart lemon icing and sprinkle with cake candies.

SWEET CEREAL PUFFS

3 egg whites	4 cups Total or Wheaties
2/3 cup sugar	

Heat oven to 325 degrees. In large mixer bowl, beat egg whites until frothy. Gradually beat in sugar; continue beating until very stiff and glossy. Fold in cereal. Drop mixture by teaspoonfuls 2 inches apart on lightly oiled baking sheet. Bake 14 to 16 minutes. Makes 3 to 4 dozen puffs.

APPLETS

8 medium firm cooking apples or 2 cups unsweetened apple pulp
½ cup cold water
2 cups white sugar
2 tablespoons unflavored gelatin
1 cup chopped walnut meats
1 tablespoon lemon juice powdered sugar

Peel and core apples; cut in small pieces. Cook in saucepan with ¼ cup of the cold water until tender. Force the cooked apples through a sieve and add white sugar. Place mixture in saucepan and cook until thick, about 30 minutes, stirring occasionally to prevent burning. Soak gelatin in remaining ¼ cup cold water, add to apple mixture, stirring until dissolved. Cool slightly by placing pan in cold water for 15–20 minutes, add walnut meats and lemon juice; mix well. Pour into flat pan to ½-inch thickness. Place in refrigerator or let stand on ice overnight. Cut in squares and roll in powdered sugar. One tablespoon cornstarch added to each cup sifted powdered sugar will prevent stickiness.

CORN FLAKE KISSES

4 cups cornflakes
1 cup sugar
1 cup raisins
1 cup nuts
½ teaspoon salt
½ teaspoon vanilla or almond extract
4 egg whites, beaten stiffly

Add sugar gradually to egg whites; fold in remaining ingredients. Drop on greased pan. Bake at 325 degrees until delicately brown.

SANDWICH FILLING SUGGESTIONS

Mayonnaise—see recipe under *Salad Dressing*

1. Hard-cooked egg white diced with dill pickle, celery and mayonnaise.
2. Old-fashioned peanut butter (unhydrogenated) and jelly.
3. Chopped chicken, celery, and pickle relish with mayonnaise.
4. Tuna fish with lemon juice, mayonnaise and grated onion.
5. Sardines, cold, or as a grilled sandwich.
6. Banana slices with peanut butter and lettuce.
7. Cottage cheese, mayonnaise and finely chopped ripe olives.
8. Cottage cheese and jelly.
9. Old-fashioned peanut butter mixed with well-drained crushed pineapple.
10. Sardines mashed and mixed with a little horseradish and mayonnaise.
11. Toasted mushroom

   Chop mushrooms, pimentoes, and onion. Cook in unsaturated oil. Sprinkle flour over mixture and stir until thick. Season with salt and pepper. Cool. Spread slices of bread with mixture. Put together in pairs and toast. Cut into strips and serve piping hot. Makes two dozen sandwiches:

1 8-oz. can mushrooms	2 tablespoons flour
1 3½-oz. can pimentoes	¾ teaspoon salt
1 small onion, diced	cayenne pepper
2 tablespoons unsaturated oil	

12. Prune-nut

1 cup chopped prunes
½ cup nuts, chopped

1 tablespoon grated orange rind
2 tablespoons brown sugar

Combine and blend well.

MISCELLANEOUS

COCOA FUDGE

2 cups sugar
½ cup skim milk
⅓ cup white syrup
3 tablespoons unsaturated oil

8 tablespoons cocoa
1 teaspoon vanilla
pinch of salt
1 cup nuts

Cook sugar, syrup, milk, salt and cocoa and oil until it forms a firm soft ball. Remove from heat, place in pan of cold water until cool. Add vanilla. Beat until creamy. Add chopped nuts and pour into greased pan. Cut when cool.

CURRIED FRUIT

1 No. 2½ can fruit, assorted
2 tablespoons unsaturated oil

½ cup sugar, white or brown
1 teaspoon curry powder

Drain fruit well, place fruit in shallow casserole. Combine other ingredients. Spoon over fruit. Bake at 325 degrees for about 1 hour. Let stand for flavor to blend. Fruit may be prepared the day in advance. Reheat before serving. This is excellent with meat.

COCOA SYRUP

1 cup cocoa	1 cup hot water
1½ cups sugar	½ inch stick cinnamon
¼ teaspoon salt	1 teaspoon vanilla

Mix cocoa, sugar and salt in sauce pan. Add hot water and stir to a paste, add cinnamon. Place over medium heat and cook to a thick syrup. Stir constantly; remove cinnamon; cool syrup. Add vanilla. Pour into a jar. Cover. Store in refrigerator. May be used on desserts, and with hot or cold skim milk as a beverage.

COCOA SAUCE

1 cup sugar	3 tablespoons cocoa
1 teaspoon flour	¾ cup water

Mix and boil and add 1 teaspoon of vanilla.

WAFFLES

1⅓ cups flour, sifted	2 egg whites, beaten stiff
2 teaspoons baking powder	1 cup skim milk
½ teaspoon salt	3 tablespoons unsaturated oil
1 teaspoon sugar	

Sift dry ingredients together. Add oil to milk. Add to dry ingredients. Fold in egg white. Makes 4 servings.

PINEAPPLE SHERBET COOLER

2 cups skim milk	1 cup drained crushed pineapple
2 cups sherbet (pineapple)	

Combine and mix in a food blender. Serve in large glasses and garnish with sprig of mint.

MILKSHAKE

¼ cup powdered skim
    milk

8 ounces low-calorie car-
    bonated creme, black
    cherry, grape or coffee
    beverages

Place powdered instant milk into blender. Pour carbon-
ated beverage over powdered skim milk. Blend at high
speed for about 2 minutes. Serve in tall glasses.

BUCKWHEAT CAKES

½ cake compressed yeast
1 cup skim milk, scalded
1 cup water
1 teaspoon salt
2 tablespoons molasses

1 cup flour
1 cup buckwheat flour
¼ teaspoon soda
¼ cup lukewarm water

Crumble yeast cake into lukewarm milk and water, add
salt, molasses and flours to make a batter as thick as
cream. Stir until free from lumps. Cover and let rise overnight at room temperature. In the morning, before baking,
stir in soda dissolved in ¼ cup lukewarm water. Pour into
small cakes and fry on hot griddle, greased. Serve with
maple syrup. Makes 20 small cakes.

CREAMY OATMEAL

1⅓ cups non-fat dry milk
    solids
4 cups water
1 teaspoon salt

2 cups Quaker Oats (quick
    or old-fashioned,
    uncooked)

Stir non-fat dry milk solids into water in a saucepan.
Bring to a boil, stirring frequently. Add salt; stir in oats.
Cook 1 minute for quick oats; 5 minutes or longer for old-
fashioned oats, stirring occasionally. Cover pan, remove

from heat and let stand a few minutes. Serve with brown sugar and skim milk. Makes 6 servings.

APPLE JELLY

2 teaspoons unflavored gelatin

2 cups unsweetened apple juice

2 tablespoons liquid sweetener

1½ tablespoons lemon juice

yellow food coloring, if desired

Soften gelatin in ½ cup of the apple juice. Bring remaining 1½ cups juice to a boil; remove from heat. Add softened gelatin, stirring to dissolve. Add liquid sweetener, lemon juice and food coloring, as desired. Bring to a rolling boil. Ladle into clean half-pint jars; seal. Keep in refrigerator. Makes 2 half-pint jars.

GRAPE JELLY

2 teaspoons unflavored gelatin

½ cup water

1½ cups unsweetened grape juice

2 tablespoons liquid sweetener

Soften gelatin in water. Bring grape juice to a boil; remove from heat. Add softened gelatin, stirring to dissolve. Add liquid sweetener. Bring to a rolling boil. Ladle into clean half-pint jars; seal. Keep in refrigerator. Makes 2 half-pint jars.

WHEAT-N-OATS

4⅓ cups water

1 teaspoon salt

2 cups Quaker Oats (quick or old-fashioned, uncooked)

½ cup wheat germ

Stir oats into briskly boiling salted water. Cook 1 minute

for quick oats, 5 minutes or longer for old-fashioned oats, stirring occasionally. Stir in wheat germ. Cover pan, remove from heat and let stand a few minutes. Serve with sugar and skim milk.

HOMEMADE NOODLES

2 egg whites, beaten
½ teaspoon salt
2 tablespoons skim milk
1 cup sifted flour
1 to 2 drops of yellow food coloring

Combine egg whites, salt, milk, and coloring. Add enough flour to make a stiff dough. Roll this to a thin sheet on floured surface. Let stand about 2 hours and then cut into thin strips. Carefully drop separated strips into boiling salted water. Cook 10 minutes. 3 cups noodles.

SPANISH NOODLE FAVORITE

1 pound lean ground meat (beef)
1 onion, chopped
1 bell pepper, chopped
1 can tomato soup
1 can whole kernel corn
1 tablespoon chili powder
1 package noodles
salt and pepper to taste

Brown the meat and drain off excess fat; add the onion and green pepper and sauté. Add the tomato soup, corn and chili powder. Cook 1 package of noodles. Add to meat mixture. Salt and pepper to taste. Bake in 350 degree oven about 1 hour.

PANCAKES

1½ cups skim milk
¼ cup safflower oil
1 egg white
2 tablespoons sugar
1½ cups Gold Medal Flour
4 teaspoons baking powder
½ teaspoon salt
syrup

Heat milk to lukewarm; stir in oil. Beat egg white with rotary beater until foamy; add sugar and beat to soft peak stage. Stir dry ingredients together; fold into oil-milk mixture in three additions, blending after each. Gently fold in egg white. Drop batter from tip of spoon onto lightly oiled heated griddle (400 degrees). When pancakes puff to ¼-inch thickness and bubbles begin to break, turn and bake on other side. Serve with syrup. Makes 18 3½-inch pancakes.

CHIFFON WAFFLES

Follow recipe for Chiffon Pancakes (above) except— bake batter in heated waffle iron. Makes 10 to 12 4½-inch waffles.

SPREAD

Delicious substitute for butter—good on toast, vegetables and for garlic bread.

1 tablespoon cornstarch	⅔ cup water
⅔ cup non-fat dry milk	2 cups safflower oil
1 teaspoon salt	few drops yellow food
1 tablespoon lemon juice	coloring

In small saucepan stir together cornstarch, non-fat dry milk and salt. Combine lemon juice and water; gradually stir into cornstarch mixture. Cook, stirring constantly, until mixture thickens and boils. Boil and stir 1 minute. Remove from heat. Cool 5 minutes. Pour into small mixer bowl. Add ½ cup oil at a time, beating after each addition. Add few drops food coloring for desired color. Cover and refrigerate. Makes 2⅔ cups.

RICE DRESSING

Try this on a flank steak that has been soaked in soy sauce for a few minutes.

4 cups cooked rice	1 teaspoon salt
1 cup bread crumbs	¼ teaspoon pepper
1 cup chopped celery	½ teaspoon sage
½ cup chopped onion	1 cup skim milk

Combine all ingredients in order. For a moistener dressing, add a little more milk.

MACARONI AND CHEESE RING

2 cups elbow macaroni	½ cup diced pimiento
¼ cup unsaturated oil and vinegar salad dressing seasoned with salt, pepper, dash of garlic powder	½ cup diced green pepper
	¼ cup finely chopped green onions or chives
2 cups uncreamed cottage cheese (you may use low-fat type)	2 tablespoons chopped parsley
	salad greens

Cook macaroni according to package directions. Drain well. Cool. Add dressing, mix well. Let stand a few minutes to marinate. Add remaining ingredients except greens. Press lightly into 9 inch ring mold. Chill several hours. Loosen sides with knife. Unmold onto chilled plate; fill center with salad greens. Serves 6–8.

CHONO COOKERY

Chono* (pronounced KO′NŌ) is a combination of dried egg whites and an artificial yolk which contains *no*

* Imitation Whole Egg Powder
  General Mills Chemicals, Inc.
  4620 W. 77th Street
  Minneapolis, Minnesota 55435

cholesterol. Safflower oil, which is highly poly-unsaturated, is used as the primary source of fat for the yolk portion. Consequently Chono is lower in saturated fat and higher in poly-unsaturated fat than dried whole eggs. The total amount of fat is also reduced in Chono. It contains approximately one-quarter as much fat as dried whole eggs. This decreases the calories per serving of Chono to about one-half the calories in an equivalent amount of dried whole eggs.

Eggs are a high quality protein food. The amino acid composition of the protein in Chono is similar to the amino acid pattern of the protein in dried whole eggs.

People wishing to control their dietary intake of cholesterol and fat can now include egg-like foods in their meals. Chono can be scrambled, prepared in omelet form, used in making French Toast, as a dip for breading and in baking and cooking. If reconstituted with water as shown on the next page, it can be used to replace beaten whole eggs in many recipes. A number of tested recipes are included on the following pages, all of which are cholesterol-free and low in saturated fat.

CHONO RECONSTITUTION GUIDE

To *measure: Dip* measuring spoon into Chono powder. *Level* off excess with a straight-edged knife or spatula.

To *reconstitute:* Measure Chono powder into a small bowl. Add cold water. Beat with rotary beater or wire whip to dissolve. For amounts of Chono and water equivalent to various numbers of eggs, see chart below.

For servings equivalent to:

	CHONO POWDER	WATER
one egg	1 tbsp. + 1 tsp. (10 gms.)	2 tbsp. + 2 tsp. (40 gms.)
two eggs	2 tbsp. + 2 tsp. (20 gms.)	⅓ cup (80 gms.)
three eggs	4 tbsp. (30 gms.)	½ cup (120 gms.)
twenty-four eggs	2 cups (240 gms.) or 1 can (8.5 oz.)	1 quart (960 gms.)

CHONOG

3 tablespoons Chono
½ cup skim milk
1 teaspoon sugar
1 cup vanilla ice milk
1 teaspoon vanilla

Measure all ingredients into blender; mix on high speed until thick and almost smooth. Sprinkle with nutmeg, if desired. 1 serving (about 10 ounces).

ORANGE-BERRY NOG

1 cup orange juice
1 cup frozen strawberries
3 tablespoons Chono
2 tablespoons non-fat milk powder
2 tablespoons sugar

Measure all ingredients into blender. Mix on low speed to blend, then on high speed until smooth. 2 servings (2 cups).

CHONO WAFFLES

¼ cup Chono
½ cup water
1½ cups buttermilk
1¾ cups all-purpose flour
2 teaspoons baking powder
1 teaspoon soda
½ teaspoon salt
½ cup shortening

Heat waffle iron. Beat Chono and water. Beat in remaining ingredients with rotary beater until smooth.

Pour batter from 1-cup measuring cup into center of hot waffle iron. Bake about 5 minutes or until steaming stops. Remove waffle carefully. Four 9-inch waffles.

CHONO PANCAKES

2 tablespoons Chono
¼ cup water
1¼ cups buttermilk
2 tablespoons safflower oil
1 cup all-purpose flour
1 tablespoon sugar
1 teaspoon baking powder
½ teapsoon soda
½ teaspoon salt

Beat Chono and water; add remaining ingredients in order listed and beat with rotary beater until smooth. Grease heated griddle if necessary. To test griddle, sprinkle with a few drops of water. If bubbles skitter around, heat is just right.

Pour batter from ¼-cup measuring cup onto hot griddle. Turn pancakes as soon as they are puffed and full of bubbles but before bubbles break. Bake other side until golden brown. Ten 4-inch pancakes.

FRENCH TOAST

3 tablespoons Chono
⅔ cup skim milk
3 slices day-old bread

2 teaspoons soft type
   margarine

Beat Chono and milk with rotary beater. Dip bread into Chono mixture. Brown both sides in margarine on *hot* griddle. Serve hot. 3 slices.

BUTTERMILK MUFFINS

1 tablespoon Chono
¼ cup water
1 cup buttermilk
¼ cup safflower oil
2 cups all-purpose flour

¼ cup sugar
2 teaspoons baking
   powder
½ teaspoon soda
1 teaspoon salt

Heat oven to 400 degrees. Grease bottoms of 15 medium muffin cups (2¾ inches in diameter). Beat Chono and water with rotary beater. Stir in buttermilk and oil. Mix in remaining ingredients *just* until flour is moistened. Batter should be lumpy.

Fill muffin cups ⅔ full. Bake 20–25 minutes or until golden brown. Immediately remove from pan. 12 muffins.

SWEET MUFFINS

1 tablespoon Chono	½ cup sugar
3 tablespoons water	2 teaspoons baking
½ cup skim milk	powder
¼ cup safflower oil	½ teaspoon salt
1½ cups all-purpose flour	

Heat oven to 400 degrees. Grease bottoms of 12 muffin cups (2¾ inches in diameter). Beat Chono and water; stir in milk and oil. Mix in remaining ingredients *just* until flour is moistened. Batter should be lumpy.

Fill muffin cups ⅔ full. Bake 20 to 25 minutes or until golden brown. Immediately remove from pan. 12 muffins.

SCRAMBLED CHONO

3 tablespoons Chono	2 teaspoons soft type margarine
⅓ cup cold water	

Beat Chono and water with rotary beater or wire whip. Heat margarine in small skillet over medium heat until just hot enough to sizzle a drop of water. Pour mixture into skillet and reduce heat to low. As mixture begins to set at bottom and sides of skillet, gently lift cooked portions with rubber spatula and fold over. AVOID CONSTANT STIRRING! Cook until mixture is thickened but still moist (about 1–2 minutes). 1 serving.

CHONO OMELET

4 tablespoons Chono	1 tablespoon soft type margarine
½ cup cold water	salt and pepper

Beat Chono and water thoroughly with rotary beater. Heat margarine in small skillet or omelet pan over medium-high heat. Pour Chono mixture into skillet. As underneath surface sets, start lifting it slightly with rubber spatula to let uncooked portion flow underneath. As soon as all of mixture seems set (top should appear moist), fold omelet into thirds. Season with salt and pepper. Serve immediately. 1 to 2 servings.

COOKED CHONNAISE

⅓ cup all-purpose flour	1 cup water
1 teaspoon sugar	¼ cup lemon juice or
1 teaspoon salt	vinegar
½ teaspoon dry mustard	1 cup safflower oil
3 tablespoons Chono	

Stir together flour, sugar, salt, mustard and Chono in medium saucepan. Stir water and lemon juice slowly into the flour mixture. Beat with rotary beater. Cook over low heat, stirring constantly, until mixture boils. Boil and stir 1 minute. Remove from heat. Pour into mixer bowl, on medium speed gradually blend in salad oil. Chill. Yields 2 cups.

CHONNAISE

1 tablespoon Chono	⅛ teaspoon white pepper
⅓ cup water	½ teaspoon salad herbs
1 teaspoon sugar	(optional)
¾ teaspoon salt	2 tablespoons lemon juice
½ teaspoon dry mustard	or vinegar
¼ teaspoon paprika	1 cup safflower oil

Have all ingredients at room temperature. Measure Chono, water, sugar, salt, mustard, paprika, pepper, salad herbs, and lemon juice into blender. Mix on low speed, slowly adding ½ cup salad oil. Beat on high speed, adding remaining salad oil *very slowly*. If necessary, stop blender and push ingredients down. Yields 1 cup.

LEMON SAUCE

1 cup sugar	6 tablespoons margarine
1 tablespoon Chono	2 to 3 teaspoons grated
⅓ cup water	lemon peel
3 tablespoons lemon juice	

Combine sugar and Chono in small saucepan. *Gradually* stir in water. Beat with rotary beater until mixture is smooth. Add lemon juice and margarine. Cook over medium heat, stirring constantly, just until mixture comes to boil. Remove from heat and stir in lemon peel. Serve warm. Yields 1⅓ cups.

Cholesterol Meal Plan Exchange List

MILK EXCHANGE—LIST 1.
PROTEIN—8 GRAMS.
CARBOHYDRATE—12 GRAMS.

Milk, powdered........	¼ cup
Buttermilk.............	1 cup
Skim milk.............	1 cup

VEGETABLES—EXCHANGE LIST 2.

GROUP A:

Insignificant carbohydrate or calories. You may eat *as much as desired* of raw vegetables. If cooked vegetable is eaten, limit amount to 1 cup.

asparagus	escarole	peppers, green or
broccoli	greens: beet,	red
brussels sprouts	chard, collard,	radishes
cabbage	dandelion, kale,	sauerkraut
cauliflower	mustard, turnip,	string beans
celery	spinach	summer squash
chicory	lettuce	tomatoes and
cucumbers	mushrooms	juice
eggplant	okra	water cress

GROUP B:
PROTEIN—2 GRAMS.
CARBOHYDRATE—7 GRAMS.

One serving equals ½ cup.

beets	onions	pumpkin	squash, winter
carrots	peas, green	rutabagas	turnips

FRUIT EXCHANGES—LIST 3.
CARBOHYDRATE—10 GRAMS.

Pour off the sauce if canned fruit. If sugar not allowed, use the diabetic canned fruit or fresh or water packed fruit.

Apple..................	1 small (2″ diam.)
Applesauce.............	½ cup
Apricots, fresh..........	2 medium
Apricots, dried..........	4 halves
Banana.................	½ small
Berries.................	1 cup
Blueberries.............	⅔ cup
Cantaloupe.............	¼ (6″ diam.)
Cherries................	10 large or 15 small
Dates..................	2
Figs, fresh..............	2 large
Figs, dried.............	1 small
Grapefruit..............	½ small
Grapefruit juice.........	½ cup
Grapes.................	12
Grape juice.............	¼ cup
Honeydew melon........	⅛ (7″ diam.)
Mango.................	½ small
Orange................	1 small
Orange juice............	½ cup
Papaya................	⅓ medium
Peach.................	1 medium
Pear...................	1 small
Apple juice.............	⅓ cup
Pineapple..............	½ cup
Pineapple juice..........	⅓ cup
Plums.................	2 medium
Prunes, dried..........	2
Raisins................	2 tablespoons
Tangerine..............	1 large
Watermelon............	1 cup

BREAD EXCHANGES—LIST 4.
PROTEIN—2 GRAMS.
CARBOHYDRATE—15 GRAMS.

Bread..........................	1 slice
biscuit, roll..................	1 (2″ diam.)
muffin......................	1 (2″ diam.)
cornbread...................	1 1½″ cube
Flour..........................	2½ tablespoons
Cereal, cooked.................	½ cup
Cereal, dry (flakes or puffed).....	¾ cup
Rice or grits, cooked...........	½ cup
Spaghetti, noodles, etc.	
cooked....................	½ cup
Crackers, graham..............	2
Crackers, saltine..............	5
Crackers, oyster...............	20
Crackers, soda.................	3
Vegetables:	
Beans (lima, navy, etc., dry)	
cooked...................	½ cup
Baked beans, no pork........	¼ cup
Peas (split, etc. dry),	
cooked...................	½ cup
Corn.......................	⅛ cup or ½ ear
Parsnips....................	⅔ cup
Potatoes, white, baked,	
boiled....................	1 (2″ diam.)
Potatoes, white, mashed.......	½ cup
Potatoes, sweet or yams.......	¼ cup
Angel Food cake...............	1½″ cube
Sherbet.......................	¼ cup

MEAT EXCHANGE—LIST 5.
PROTEIN—7 GRAMS.
FAT—5 GRAMS.

Lean Group—use these meats at least 5 times per week
    veal, liver, turkey, chicken, kidney........ 1 slice (3" x 2" x ½")
Fatty Group—use these meats not more than 3 times per week
    duck, tongue, beef, lamb, pork, ham,
      Canadian bacon...................... 1 slice
Fish Group—use fish at least 5 times per week
    codfish, mackerel, pike, etc.............. 1 slice (2" x 2" x 1")
    salmon, tuna, crab, lobster.............. ¼ cup
    oysters, shrimp, clams.................. 5 small
    sardines............................... 3 medium
Dry curd cottage cheese................... ¼ cup
Egg—according to allowance.............. 1
Peanut butter, unhydrogenated............. 2 tablespoons

FAT EXCHANGE—LIST 6.
FAT—5 GRAMS.

Soft type margarine oil spread.............. 1 teaspoon
French Dressing—made with unsaturated oil.. 1 tablespoon
Mayonnaise—made without egg yolk........ 1 teaspoon
Unsaturated oil........................... 1 teaspoon
Nuts..................................... 6 small
Olives.................................... 5 small
Avocado:................................. ⅛ (4" diam.)
Sunflower seeds, hulled................... ¼ oz. (½ tablespoon)
Sesame seeds............................. ¼ oz. (½ tablespoon)

Common Artificial Sweeteners

SUCARYL

⅛ teaspoon = 1 teaspoon sugar
⅜ teaspoon = 1 tablespoon sugar
1 teaspoon = 8 teaspoons sugar
1½ teaspoons = ¼ cup sugar
2 teaspoons = ⅓ cup sugar
1 tablespoon = ½ cup sugar
2 tablespoons = 1 cup sugar

SWEET 10 (LIQUID)

⅛ teaspoon = 1 teaspoon sugar
¼ teaspoon = 2 teaspoons sugar
⅜ teaspoon = 1 tablespoon sugar
1½ teaspoons = ¼ cup sugar
2 teaspoons = ⅓ cup sugar
1 tablespoon = ½ cup sugar

SPRINKLE SWEET

1 teaspoon = 1 teaspoon sugar
2 teaspoons = 2 teaspoons sugar
1 tablespoon = 1 tablespoon sugar
¼ cup = ¼ cup sugar
⅓ cup = ⅓ cup sugar
½ cup = ½ cup sugar

SWEET & LOW

1 packet = 2 teaspoons sugar
3 packets = 2 tablespoons sugar
6 packets = ¼ cup sugar
12 packets = ½ cup sugar
24 packets = 1 cup sugar
3 teaspoons = ½ cup sugar
6 teaspoons = 1 cup sugar

SACCHARIN

¼ Grain = 1 teaspoon sugar

Substitutions

FOR:	USE:
1 cup sifted all-purpose flour	1 cup plus 2 tablespoons sifted cake flour
1 cup sifted cake flour	1 cup minus 2 tablespoons sifted all-purpose flour
1 tablespoon cornstarch (for thickening)	2 tablespoons flour
1 teaspoon baking powder	¼ teaspoon soda plus ½ teaspoon cream of tartar
1 cup skim milk	4 tablespoons powdered milk plus 1 cup water
1 cup skim milk	1 cup sour milk or buttermilk plus $\frac{1}{2}$ teaspoon soda (decrease baking powder 2 teaspoons)
1 cup sour milk or buttermilk	1 cup fresh skim milk with 1 tablespoon lemon juice or vinegar stirred in

FOR:	USE:
1 square unsweetened chocolate (1 ounce)	3 to 4 tablespoons cocoa plus 1 tablespoon shortening
1 cup honey	¾ cup sugar plus ¼ cup liquid
1 cup sugar	1 cup honey or syrup and reduce liquid in recipe ¼ cup (in cakes substitute honey for only ½ the sugar)
1 cup brown sugar (firmly packed)	1 cup granulated sugar
1 cup sugar (½ pound)	1⅙ cups powdered sugar
1 cup sugar	1¾ cups confectioners' (sifted)
1 cup canned tomatoes	about 1⅓ cups cut up fresh tomatoes, simmered 10 minutes
1 whole egg	1 tablespoon and 1 teaspoon "chono" plus 5 teaspoons water to reconstitute

REFERENCES OF INTEREST

(Abbreviated Bibliography)

1. Turner, Dorothea: *Handbook of Diet Therapy*, The University of Chicago Press, Chicago 37, Illinois, 3rd edition, 1959. $5.00.
2. Keys, Ancel and Margaret: *Eat Well and Stay Well.* Doubleday and Company, Inc., Garden City, New York, 1959. $3.85.
3. Payne, A. S. and Callahan, Dorothy: *Low-Sodium, Fat-Controlled Cookbook.* Little Brown Publishing Company, Boston, 1960. $4.75.
4. Revell, Dorothy: *Dietary Control of Hypercholesteremia.* Charles C. Thomas, Publisher, Springfield, Illinois, 1962. $4.50.
5. Revell, Dorothy: *How Diabetics Can Eat Wisely.* T. S. Denison and Company, Inc., Minneapolis, Minn. $3.95.
6. Stead and Warren: *Low Fat Cookery.* Blakiston Division, McGraw-Hill Book Company, New York, 1959. $4.50.
7. Gofman, John; Nichols, Alex V. and Dobbin, E. Virginia: *Dietary Prevention and Treatment of Heart Disease.* G. P. Putnam's Sons, New York, 1958. $3.95.

8. *Controlled Fat Menu Plan*, Moderately High in Unsaturated Fats. California Heart Association, 1428 Bush Street, San Francisco 9, California, June, 1960.

9. Zugibe, Frederick T., *Eat, Drink, and Lower Your Cholesterol*, McGraw-Hill, $4.95.

10. Gofman, John W., M.D., *Low Fat, Low Cholesterol Diet*, Doubleday & Co., $4.50.

11. Morrison, Lester, M.D., *Low Fat Way to Health & Longer Life*, Prentice-Hall, Inc., $4.95.

12. Revell, Dorothy, *Gourmet Recipes for Diabetics*, Charles C. Thomas, Publisher, Springfield, Illinois, 1971. $9.50.

Recipe Index

Appetizers

Bac*-Os *Cottage Cheese* Diet Dip, 59
Blender *Cheese* Dip, 59
Cottage Cheese Spread, 60
Crab Dip, 58
Curry Spread, 60
Green Onion Dip, 60
Meat Spread, 57
Spiced Pickle *Shrimp,* 58
Stuffed *Celery Sticks,* 60
Stuffed *Egg Whites,* 59
Tuna Canapes, 58
Tuna Spread, 60

Soups

Corn Soup, 63
Crab Soup, 61
Fish Chowder, 62
Potato Soup, 62
Potato Ham Chowder, 61
Split *Pea Soup,* 62
Vegetable Bouillon, 63

Breads

Biscuits I, 63
Biscuits II, 64
Biscuits, *Sweet Potato,* 68
Breakfast Puffs, 68
Buttermilk Muffins, 65
Carrot-Orange Bread, 65
Cinnamon Muffins, 69
Graham Bread, 67
Oatmeal Bread, 66
Pineapple Biscuits, 67
Spicy Twists, 66
Sweet Potato Biscuits, 68
White *Corn Bread,* 65

Sauces

Barbecue, 69
Basic *Cream Sauce* With Dry Skim Milk, 74
Benedictine Sauce, 112
Blueberry Sauce, 70
Bourbon Marinade for Beef, 71
Brandy Cream, 123
Brown Gravy, 70
Chono *Lemon Sauce,* 149
Cocoa Sauce, 138
Curry Sauce, 92
Custard Sauce, 72
Fish Cocktail Sauce, 73
Foaming *Pudding Sauce,* 110
Low Calorie *Lemon Sauce,* 69
(Mornay Sauce)
Mint Sauce, 84
Mustard Marinade for Beef, 73
Orange Sauce, 112

Parsley Sauce, 83
Piquant Sauce, 79
Port Sauce for Meat, 70
Spaghetti Sauce With Meat, 72
Sweet-Sour Bar-B-Que Sauce, 72
Tartar Spread, 71
Teriyaki Sauce, 73
White Sauce, 71

Meats

Baked Spiced *Pork Chops*, 90
Beef With Mushrooms, 86
Beef Stew, 80
Leg of *Lamb With Mint Sauce*, 84
Meat Loaf, 75
Oven-Baked Spanish *Pork Chop*, 75
Pork, Oriental Style, 86
Steak, Diane, 87
Stuffed *Pork Chop*, 85
Veal à la Marengo, 77
Veal or Beef Tomato, 87

Fish

Baked With Piquant Sauce, 79
Baked *Salmon*, 74
Braised, Portuguese, 78
Cod in White Wine, 84
Crab Meat Pancakes, 76
and *Potato Casserole*, 91
Fillets, 75
and *Noodles*, 76
With Wine and Tomatoes, 83
Lobster Genovese, 92
Red Snapper, 77
Salmon Steak, 84

Shrimp With Curry Sauce, 92
Sole in Parsley Sauce, 83

Poultry

Chicken, Baked, With Apricots, 88
Chicken à la Marengo, 77
Chicken Cacciatora, 89
Chicken Casserole, 82
Chicken Chow Mein (American Style), 90
Chicken with Madeira, 82
Chicken Jubilee, 81
Chicken Curried, with Papaya, 79
Chicken Salad, Hot, 99
Chicken International Dateline, 81
Chicken Oven Baked in Wine, 74
Skillet Pineapple *Chicken*, 91
Turkey Divan, 88
Duck à l' Orange, Wild, 85

Salad Dressings

Avocado, 95
Creamy *Mayonnaise*, 95
Curry, 94
French, 96
Honey, 95
Mustard, 100
Never-Fail *Mayonnaise*, 92
Oil and Vinegar, 93
Potato *Mayonnaise*, 93
Russian, 93
Sesame Seed, 93
Sunshine, 94
Sweet, 96
Sweet-Sour, 94
Zero, 94

Salads

Avocado and Tuna, 97
Chinese Chicken, 97
Cole Slaw, 100
Cucumbers in Vinaigrette, 99
Chicken, Hot, 99
Garden Relish, 99
Fruit Medley, 98
Molded Cottage Cheese, 96
Pineapple Carrot, 98
Fish With Vegetables, Raw, 97
Suggestions, 100–1

Cakes

Bonnie, 104
Buttercup, 104
Cherry Angel Food, 106
Cinnamon Coffee, 106
Cocoa, 108
Eggless Fruit, 107
Gingerbread, 105
Hawaiian, 108
Ice Water, 103
Lady Baltimore, 101
Mayonnaise, 101
Old-fashioned Gingerbread, 105
Poppy Seed White, 107
Strawberry Shortcake, 121
White, 102

Frosting and Toppings

Apple Snow, 110
Cocoa, 111
Fluffy Apricot, 109
Fluffy White, 102
Foaming Pudding Sauce, 110
Fresh Strawberry Icing, 109
Fruit Filling, 102
Harvest Moon, 109
Honey, 110
Low Calorie Whipped Topping, 111
Low Calorie Orange Whipped Topping, 111
Mocha Icing, 109
Pineapple Filling, 103
Seven Minute Icing, 103
White Icing, 110

Desserts

Ambrosia Chiffon Pie, 119
Angel Pie, 115
Apple Betty, 115
Apple Charlotte, 117
Apple Dessert, 122
Apple-Nut Pudding, 116
Baked Alaska, 120
Baked Peaches, 117
Banana Crisp, 122
Banana Souffle, 120
Brandy Cream, 123
Brownies, 113
Cocoa Pudding, 116
Cherry Frappé, 119
Cracker Pie, 119
Cranberry Ice, 113
Date Delight, 113
Date-Nut Torte, 117
Green Gage Plum Ice, 115
Jello Sherbet, 113
Lemon Sherbet, 123
Fruit Mapley Baked, 123
Melon Parfaits, 121
Pie Crust, 118
Plum Pudding, uncooked, 112
Prune Souffle, 114
Raspberry Whip, 118
Rebecca Pudding, 118
Ritz Delight, 114

Spicy *Fruit Pudding*, 116
Spring Parfait, 121
Strawberry Short Cake, 121
Strawberry Souffle, 120
Strawberry Supreme, 122

Vegetables

Asparagus Par Excellence, 125
Baked *Eggplant*, 125
Baked *Tomatoes Supreme*, 127
Cabbage with Caraway Seeds, 124
Carrots Medley, 127
Chinese Peas, 128
Curried *Potatoes*, 128
Curried *Spinach*, 126
Fluffy *Acorn Squash*, 126
Maple *Sweet Potatoes*, 127
Okra and Tomatoes, 126
Peas and Celery, 124
Sweet-Sour *Zucchini*, 128

Cookies

Almond-Date, 131
Applets, 135
Chewy *Oatmeal*, 131
Chinese Chews, 129
Cornflake Kisses, 135
Crisp *Ginger Snaps*, 130
Fruit Bites, unbaked, 129
Ginger Snaps, 131
Jordon Specials, 134
Lemon Wafers, 133
Marguerites, 134
Oat Squares, 133
Oatmeal Cookies, 132
Oatmeal Cocoa, unbaked, 129
Pecan Kisses, 130

Sesame Cookies, 133
Stir-N-Drop *Sugar*, 132
Sweet *Cereal Puffs*, 134
Whiskey Balls, unbaked, 130

Sandwich Filling Suggestions

Banana Slices, 136
Chopped *Chicken*, 136
Cottage Cheese and Jelly, 136
Cottage Cheese and Olives, 136
Hard Cooked *Egg Whites and Pickles*, 136
Old-fashioned *Peanut Butter and Jelly*, 136
Old-fashioned *Peanut Butter and Pineapple*, 136
Prune-Nut Sandwich, 137
Toasted *Mushroom*, 136
Tuna Fish and Onion, 136
Sardine, 136
Sardine and Horseradish, 136

Miscellaneous

Apple Jelly, 140
Buckwheat Cakes, 139
Chiffon Waffles, 142
Cocoa Fudge, 137
Cocoa Sauce, 138
Cocoa Syrup, 138
Creamy *Oatmeal*, 139
Curried *Fruit*, 137
Grape Jelly, 140
Homemade *Noodles*, 141
Macaroni and Cheese Ring, 143
Milkshake, 139
Pancakes, 141
Pineapple Sherbet Cooler, 138
Rice Dressing, 142

164

Spanish *Noodles*, 141
Bread Spread, 142
Waffles, 138
Wheat-N-Oats, 140

Chono Cookery

Buttermilk Muffins, 146
Chonog, 145

Chonnaise, 148
Chonnaise, Cooked, 148
French Toast, 146
Lemon Sauce, 149
Omelet, 147
Orange-Berry Nog, 145
Pancakes, 145
Scrambled Chono, 147
Sweet Muffins, 147
Waffles, 145

INDEX

Acorn Squash, Fluffy, 126
Almond-Date Cookies, 131
Ambrosia Chiffon Pie, 119
Angel Pie, 115
Appetizers
  Celery Sticks, Stuffed, 60
  Cheese Dip, Blender, 59
  Cottage Cheese Diet Dip, Bac*-Os, 59
  Cottage Cheese Spread, 60
  Crab Dip, 58
  Curry Spread, 60
  Egg Whites, Stuffed, 59
  Meat Spread, 57
  Onion Dip, Green, 60
  Shrimp, Spiced Pickled, 58
  Tuna Canapes, 58
  Tuna Spread, 60
Apple Betty, 115
Apple Charlotte, 117
Apple Dessert, 122
Apple Jelly, 140
Apple-Nut Pudding, 116
Apple Snow Frosting, 110
Applets, 135
Apricot Sauce, Fluffy, 109
Asparagus Par Excellence, 125
Avocado Dressing, 95
Avocado and Tuna Salad, 97

Baked Alaska, 120

Banana Crisp, 122
Banana Slices, Sandwich Filling, 136
Banana Soufflé, 120
Barbecue Sauce, 69
Bar-B-Q Sauce, Sweet-Sour, 72
Beef with Mushrooms, 86
Beef Stew, 80
Beef Tomato, Veal or, 87
Benedictine Sauce, 112
Biscuits I, 63
Biscuits II, 64
Blueberry Sauce, 70
Bonnie Cake, 104
Bourbon Marinade for Beef, 71
Brandy Cream, 123
Bread Spread, 142
Breads
  Biscuits I, 63
  Biscuits II, 64
  Breakfast Puffs, 68
  Buttermilk Muffins, 65
  Carrot-Orange Bread, 65
  Cinnamon Muffins, 69
  Corn Bread, White, 65
  Graham Bread, 67
  Oatmeal Bread, 66
  Pineapple Biscuits, 67
  Spicy Twists, 66
  Sweet Potato Biscuits, 68
Breakfast Puffs, 68

Brown Gravy, 70
Brownies, 113
Buckwheat Cakes, 139
Buttercup Cake, 104
Buttermilk Muffins, 65
Buttermilk Muffins, Chono, 146

Cabbage with Caraway Seeds, 124
Cakes *See also* Desserts
    Bonnie, 104
    Buttercup, 104
    Cherry Angel Food, 106
    Cinnamon Coffee Cake, 106
    Cocoa, 108
    Eggless Fruit, 107
    Gingerbread, 105
    Gingerbread, Old-fashioned, 105
    Hawaiian, 108
    Ice Water, 103
    Lady Baltimore, 101
    Mayonnaise, 101
    Poppy Seed White, 107
    Strawberry Shortcake, 121
    White, 102
Carrot-Orange Bread, 65
Carrots Medley, 127
Celery Sticks, Stuffed, 60
Cereal Puffs, Sweet, 134
Cheese Dip, Blender, 59
Cherry Angel Food Cake, 106
Cherry Frappé, 119
Chicken, Baked, with Apricots, 88
Chicken Cacciatora, 89
Chicken Casserole, 82
Chicken, Chinese, Salad, 97
Chicken, Chopped, Sandwich Filling, 136

Chicken Chow Mein (American style), 90
Chicken, Curried, with Papaya, 79
Chicken, International Dateline, 81
Chicken Jubilee, 81
Chicken with Madeira, 82
Chicken à la Marengo, 77
Chicken, Oven-Baked, in Wine, 74
Chicken Salad, Hot, 99
Chicken, Skillet Pineapple, 91
Chiffon Waffles, 142
Chinese Chews, 129
Chono Cookery
    Chonnaise, 148
    Chonnaise, Cooked, 148
    Chono, Scrambled, 147
    Chonog, 145
    French Toast, 146
    Lemon Sauce, 149
    Muffins, Buttermilk, 146
    Muffins, Sweet, 147
    Omelet, 147
    Orange-Berry Nog, 145
    Pancakes, 145
    Waffles, 145
Cinnamon Coffee Cake, 106
Cinnamon Muffins, 69
Cocoa Cake, 108
Cocoa Frosting, 111
Cocoa Fudge, 137
Cocoa Pudding, 116
Cocoa Sauce, 138
Cocoa Syrup, 138
Cod in White Wine, 84
Cole Slaw, 100
Cookies *See also* Desserts
    Almond-Date, 131
    Applets, 135
    Cereal Puffs, Sweet, 134
    Chinese Chews, 129

168

Cornflake Kisses, 135
Fruit Bites, Unbaked, 129
Ginger Snaps, 131
Ginger Snaps, Crisp, 130
Jordan Specials, 134
Lemon Wafers, 133
Marguerites, 134
Oatmeal Cocoa, Unbaked, 129
Oatmeal, 132
Oatmeal, Chewy, 131
Oat Squares, 133
Pecan Kisses, 130
Sesame, 133
Sugar, Stir-N-Drop, 132
Whiskey Balls, Unbaked, 130
Corn Bread, White, 65
Cornflake Kisses, 135
Corn Soup, 63
Cottage Cheese Diet Dip, Bac*-Os, 59
Cottage Cheese and Jelly, Sandwich Filling, 136
Cottage Cheese, Molded, Salad, 96
Cottage Cheese and Olives, Sandwich Filling, 136
Cottage Cheese Spread, 60
Crab Dip, 58
Crab Meat Pancakes, 76
Crab Soup, 61
Cracker Pie, 119
Cranberry Ice, 113
Cream Sauce, Basic, With Dry Skim Milk, 74
Cucumbers in Vinaigrette, 99
Curried Fruit, 137
Curried Potatoes, 128
Curried Spinach, 126
Curry Dressing, 94
Curry Sauce, 92
Curry Spread, 60

Custard Sauce, 72

Date Delight, 113
Date-Nut Torte, 117
Desserts
    Ambrosia Chiffon Pie, 119
    Angel Pie, 115
    Apple Betty, 115
    Apple Charlotte, 117
    Apple Dessert, 122
    Apple-Nut Pudding, 116
    Baked Alaska, 120
    Banana Crisp, 122
    Banana Soufflé, 120
    Brandy Cream, 123
    Brownies, 113
    Cocoa Pudding, 116
    Cherry Frappé, 119
    Cracker Pie, 119
    Cranberry Ice, 113
    Date Delight, 113
    Date-Nut Torte, 117
    Fruit, Mapley Baked, 123
    Fruit Pudding, Spicy, 116
    Jello Sherbet, 113
    Lemon Sherbet, 123
    Melon Parfaits, 121
    Peaches, Baked, 117
    Pie Crust, 118
    Plum Ice, Green Gage, 115
    Plum Pudding, Uncooked, 112
    Prune Soufflé, 114
    Raspberry Whip, 118
    Rebecca Pudding, 118
    Ritz Delight, 114
    Spring Parfait, 121
    Strawberry Shortcake, 121
    Strawbery Soufflé, 120
    Strawberry Supreme, 122
Dressings
    Avocado, 95

169

Curry, 94
French, 96
Honey, 95
Mayonnaise, Creamy, 95
Mayonnaise, Never-Fail, 92
Mayonnaise, Potato, 93
Mustard, 100
Oil and Vinegar, 93
Russian, 93
Sesame Seed, 93
Sunshine, 94
Sweet, 96
Sweet-Sour, 94
Zero, 94
Duck, Wild, à l'Orange, 85

Eggless Fruit Cake, 107
Eggplant, Baked, 125
Egg Whites, Hard Cooked, and Pickles, Sandwich Filling, 136
Egg Whites, Stuffed, 59

Fish, Baked, with Piquant Sauce, 79
Fish, Braised, Portuguese, 78
Fish Chowder, 62
Fish Cocktail Sauce, 73
Fish Fillets, 75
Fish and Noodles, 76
Fish and Potato Casserole, 91
Fish, Raw, with Vegetables, 97
Fish with Wine and Tomatoes, 83
French Dressing, 96
French Toast, Chono, 146
Frostings, Fillings and Toppings
    Apple Snow Frosting, 110

Apricot Sauce, Fluffy, 109
Cocoa Frosting, 111
Fruit Filling, 102
Harvest Moon Frosting, 109
Honey Frosting, 110
Mocha Icing, 109
Pineapple Filling, 103
Pudding Sauce, Foaming, 110
Seven Minute Icing, 103
Strawberry Icing, Fresh, 109
White Frosting, Fluffy, 102
Whipped Topping, Low Calorie, 111
Whipped Topping, Low Calorie Orange, 111
White Icing, 110
Fruit Bites, Unbaked, 129
Fruit Cake, Eggless, 107
Fruit, Curried, 137
Fruit Filling, 102
Fruit, Mapley Baked, 123
Fruit Medley, 98
Fruit Pudding, Spicy, 116

Garden Relish Salad, 99
Gingerbread Cake, 105
Gingerbread, Old-Fashioned, 105
Ginger Snaps, 131
Ginger Snaps, Crisp, 130
Graham Bread, 67
Grape Jelly, 140

Harvest Moon Frosting, 109
Hawaiian Cake, 108
Honey Dressing, 95
Honey Frosting, 110

Ice Water Cake, 103

Jello Sherbet, 113
Jelly, Apple, 140
Jelly Grape, 140
Jordan Specials, 134

Lady Baltimore Cake, 101
Lamb, Leg of, with Mint Sauce, 84
Lemon Sauce, Chono, 149
Lemon Sauce, Low Calorie, 69
Lemon Sherbet, 123
Lemon Wafers, 133
Lobster Genovese, 92

Macaroni and Cheese Ring, 143
Mapley Baked Fruit, 123
Marguerites, 134
Mayonnaise Cake, 101
Mayonnaise, Creamy, 95
Mayonnaise, Never-Fail, 92
Mayonnaise, Potato, 93
Meats
  Beef Tomato, Veal or, 87
  Beef with Mushrooms, 86
  Beef Stew, 80
  Lamb, Leg of, with Mint Sauce, 84
  Meat Loaf, 75
  Pork Chops, Baked Spiced, 90
  Pork Chops, Oven-Baked Spanish, 75
  Pork Chops, Stuffed, 85
  Pork, Oriental Style, 86
  Steak Diane, 87
  Veal à la Marengo, 77

Veal or Beef Tomato, 87
Meat Loaf, 75
Meat Spread, 57
Melon Parfaits, 121
Milk Shake, 139
Mint Sauce, 84
Mocha Icing, 109
Muffins, Sweet, Chono, 147
  See also Breads
Mushroom, Toasted, Sandwich Filling, 136
Mustard Dressing, 100
Mustard Marinade for Beef, 73

Noodles, Homemade, 141
Noodles, Spanish, 141

Oatmeal Bread, 66
Oatmeal Cocoa, Cookies, Unbaked, 129
Oatmeal Cookies, 132
Oatmeal Cookies, Chewy, 131
Oatmeal, Creamy, 139
Oat Squares, 133
Oil and Vinegar Dressing, 93
Okra and Tomatoes, 126
Omelet, Chono, 147
Onion Dip, Green, 60
Orange-Berry Nog, Chono, 145
Orange Sauce, 112

Pancakes and Waffles
  Buckwheat Cakes, 139
  Chono Pancakes, 145
  Chono Waffles, 145
  Chiffon Waffles, 142
  Pancakes, 141
  Waffles, 138

Parsley Sauce, 83
Peaches, Baked, 117
Peanut Butter and Jelly, Old-Fashioned, Sandwich Filling, 136
Peanut Butter and Pineapple, Old Fashioned, Sandwich Filling, 136
Pea Soup, Split, 62
Peas and Celery, 124
Peas, Chinese, 128
Pecan Kisses, 130
Pie Crust, 118
Pies *See* Desserts
Pineapple Biscuits, 67
Pineapple Carrot Salad, 98
Pineapple Filling, 103
Pineapple Sherbet Cooler, 138
Piquant Sauce, 79
Plum Ice, Green Gage, 115
Plum Pudding, Uncooked, 112
Poppy Seed White Cake, 107
Pork Chops, Baked, Spiced, 90
Pork Chops, Oven-Baked Spanish, 75
Pork Chops, Stuffed, 85
Pork, Oriental Style, 86
Port Sauce for Meat, 70
Potato Ham Chowder, 61
Potato Soup, 62
Potatoes, Curried, 128
Poultry
  Chicken, Baked, with Apricots, 88
  Chicken Cacciatora, 89
  Chicken Casserole, 82
  Chicken Chow Mein (American Style), 90
  Chicken, Curried, with Papaya, 79

Chicken, International Dateline, 81
Chicken Jubilee, 81
Chicken with Madeira, 82
Chicken à la Marengo, 77
Chicken, Oven Baked, in Wine, 74
Chicken Salad, Hot, 99
Chicken, Skillet Pineapple, 91
  Duck, Wild, à l'Orange, 85
  Turkey Divan, 88
Prune Nut Sandwich, 137
Prune Soufflé, 114
Puddings *See* Desserts
Pudding Sauce, Foaming, 110

Raspberry Whip, 118
Rebecca Pudding, 118
Red Snapper, 77
Rice Dressing, 142
Ritz Delight, 114
Russian Dressing, 93

Salads
  Avocado and Tuna, 97
  Chicken, Chinese, 97
  Chicken, Hot, 99
  Cole Slaw, 100
  Cottage Cheese, Molded, 96
  Cucumbers in Vinaigrette, 99
  Fish, Raw, with Vegetables, 97
  Fruit Medley, 98
  Garden Relish, 99
  Pineapple Carrot, 98
  Salad Suggestions, 100–1
Salmon, Baked, 74
Salmon Steak, 84

Sandwich Fillings
  Banana slices, 136
  Chicken, Chopped, 136
  Cottage Cheese and Jelly, 136
  Cottage Cheese and Olives, 136
  Egg Whites, Hard-Cooked and Pickles, 136
  Mushroom, Toasted, 136
  Peanut Butter and Jelly, Old Fashioned, 136
  Peanut Butter and Pineapple, Old Fashioned, 136
  Prune Nut, 137
  Sardines, 136
  Sardine and Horseradish, 136
  Tuna Fish and Onion, 136
Sardine Sandwich Filling, 136
Sardine and Horseradish Sandwich Filling, 136
Sauces
  Barbecue, 69
  Bar-B-Q, Sweet-Sour, 72
  Benedictine, 112
  Blueberry, 70
  Bourbon Marinade for Beef, 71
  Brandy Cream, 123
  Brown Gravy, 70
  Cocoa, 138
  Cream, Basic, with Dry Skim Milk, 74
  Curry, 92
  Custard, 72
  Fish Cocktail, 73
  Lemon, Chono, 149
  Lemon, Low Calorie, 69
  Mint, 84
  Mustard Marinade for Beef, 73
  Orange, 112

  Parsley, 83
  Piquant, 79
  Port, for Meat, 70
  Pudding, Foaming, 110
  Spaghetti, with Meat, 72
  Tartar Spread, 71
  Teriyaki, 73
  White, 71
Seafood
  Cod in White Wine, 84
  Crab Meat Pancakes, 76
  Fish, with Piquant Sauce, Baked, 79
  Fish, Braised, Portuguese, 78
  Fish Fillets, 75
  Fish and Noodles, 76
  Fish and Potato Casserole, 91
  Fish with Wine and Tomatoes, 83
  Lobster Genovese, 92
  Red Snapper, 77
  Salmon, Baked, 74
  Salmon Steak, 84
  Shrimp with Curry Sauce, 92
  Sole, Baked, in Parsley Sauce, 83
Sesame Cookies, 133
Sesame Seed Dressing, 93
Seven Minute Icing, 103
Shrimp with Curry Sauce, 92
Shrimp, Spiced Pickled, 58
Sole, Baked, in Parsley Sauce, 83
Soups
  Corn, 63
  Crab, 61
  Fish Chowder, 62
  Pea, Split, 62
  Potato Ham Chowder, 61
  Potato, 62

Vegetable Bouillon, 63
Spaghetti Sauce with Meat, 72
Spicy Twists, 66
Spinach, Curried, 126
Spring Parfait, 121
Steak Diane, 87
Strawberry Icing, Fresh, 109
Strawberry Shortcake, 121
Strawberry Soufflé, 120
Strawberry Supreme, 122
Sugar Cookies, Stir-N-Drop, 132
Sunshine Dressing, 94
Sweet Dressing, 96
Sweet Potato Biscuits, 68
Sweet Potatoes, Maple, 127
Sweet-Sour Dressing, 94

Tartar Spread, 71
Teriyaki Sauce, 73
Tomatoes Supreme, Baked, 127
Tuna Canapes, 58
Tuna Fish and Onion, Sandwich Filling, 136
Tuna Spread, 60
Turkey Divan, 88

Veal or Beef Tomato, 87
Veal à la Marengo, 77
Vegetables
  Acorn Squash, Fluffy, 126
  Asparagus Par Excellence, 125
  Cabbage with Caraway Seeds, 124
  Carrots Medley, 127
  Eggplant, Baked, 125
  Okra and Tomatoes, 126
  Peas and Celery, 124
  Peas, Chinese, 128
  Potatoes, Curried, 128
  Spinach, Curried, 126
  Sweet Potatoes, Maple, 127
  Tomatoes Supreme, Baked, 127
  Zucchini, Sweet-Sour, 128
Vegetable Bouillon, 63

Waffles, 138
Waffles, Chono, 145
Waffles, Chiffon, 142
Wheat-N-Oats, 140
Whipped Topping, Low Calorie, 111
Whipped Topping, Low Calorie Orange, 111
Whiskey Balls, Unbaked, 130
White Cake, 102
White Frosting, Fluffy, 102
White Icing, 110
White Sauce, 71

Zero Dressing, 94
Zucchini, Sweet-Sour, 128